PLANT BASED COOKBOOK FOR BEGINNERS

Plant-Based Prep: Wholesome Recipes for Boosting Mental Focus and Energizing Your Day

DANIEL EDWARDS

TABLE OF CONTENTS

Introduction 4

Chapter 1: Introduction to Plant-Based Eating 7

Chapter 2: Understanding Nutritional Needs 48

Chapter 3: Breakfast Boosters 93

Chapter 4: Midday Meals for Sustained Energy 163

Chapter 5: Healthy Plant-Based Snacks 244

Chapter 6: Creative Dinner Ideas 293

Chapter 7: Sweet Treats without the Guilt. 316

Conclusion 340

Introduction

Making the switch to a plant-based diet can seem daunting at first, but the benefits are plentiful - from increased energy and mental clarity to reduced inflammation and lower risk of chronic diseases. This cookbook is designed to make that transition smooth and delicious for anyone looking to embrace a plant-based lifestyle, even if it's your first time.

The carefully crafted recipes in this book put clean, nutrient-dense whole foods at the forefront, helping to power your mind and body from morning to night. You'll find invigorating breakfasts like Blueberry Omega-

3 Waffles to kickstart your day, energizing lunches such as the Curried Cauliflower Veggie Wraps to beat the afternoon slump, and hearty dinners like Lentil Quinoa Burgers that will satisfy and nourish.

Beyond just recipes, you'll also discover helpful tips for stocking your plant-based pantry, simple food prep tricks to save time, and ways to boost the nutritional punch of each dish. Every recipe utilizes normal kitchen equipment and easy-to-find ingredients so you can start cooking wholesome, energizing meals right away.

Whether your goal is to sharpen your focus at work or school, enhance athletic performance, or just feel your best every day, the diverse array of flavors and nutrient-rich recipes in this book will inspire you on your plant-based journey to vitality. Let's get cooking!

Chapter 1

Introduction to Plant-Based Eating

What is plant-based eating?

In an era where health and environmental consciousness are becoming increasingly paramount, the concept of plant-based eating has gained significant traction. This dietary approach, which emphasizes the consumption of plant-derived foods, offers a multitude of benefits that extend far beyond mere sustenance. By embracing the abundance of nature's bounty, individuals can embark on a journey towards improved well-being, environmental stewardship, and ethical considerations.

At its core, plant-based eating is a dietary philosophy that prioritizes the consumption of fruits, vegetables, whole grains, legumes, nuts, and seeds. While some adherents adopt a strict vegan lifestyle, eliminating all animal products, others opt for a more flexible approach, incorporating modest amounts of dairy, eggs, or even occasional servings of ethically-sourced meat or seafood. Ultimately, the fundamental principle lies in deriving the majority of one's nutritional intake from plant-based sources.

One of the most compelling arguments in favor of plant-based eating is its profound impact on personal health. Numerous scientific studies have consistently demonstrated that a diet rich in plant-based foods is associated with a reduced risk of chronic diseases, including heart disease, certain types of cancer, and type 2 diabetes. This correlation can be attributed to the abundance of essential nutrients, such as fiber, antioxidants, and phytochemicals, found in plant-based foods.

Fiber, a crucial component of plant-based diets, plays a vital role in promoting digestive health and regulating blood sugar levels. Antioxidants, which are abundant in fruits and vegetables, combat oxidative stress and inflammation, thereby reducing the risk of various chronic conditions. Furthermore, phytochemicals, the natural compounds found in plants, possess potent anti-inflammatory and anti-cancer properties, fortifying the body's defenses against disease.

Beyond physical health, plant-based eating can also contribute to mental well-being. Studies have indicated that individuals following a plant-based diet tend to experience lower rates of depression and anxiety, potentially due to the presence of mood-boosting nutrients like omega-3 fatty acids, vitamin B12, and folate. Additionally, the consumption of whole, unprocessed plant-based foods can promote a sense of vitality and overall well-being, enhancing one's quality of life.

Environmental concerns are another driving force behind the growing popularity of plant-based eating. The production of animal-based foods, particularly meat and dairy, has a significantly higher environmental impact compared to plant-based alternatives. Animal agriculture is a major contributor to greenhouse gas emissions, land degradation, water pollution, and deforestation. By shifting towards a more plant-based diet, individuals can reduce their carbon footprint and contribute to a more sustainable future for our planet.

Moreover, the ethical considerations associated with plant-based eating cannot be overlooked. Many individuals choose to adopt this lifestyle out of a desire to reduce animal suffering and promote more humane practices. Factory farming, which is prevalent in the modern food industry, often subjects animals to inhumane living conditions and cruel treatment. By opting for plant-based alternatives, individuals can make a conscious choice to align their values with their dietary habits.

Despite the numerous benefits of plant-based eating, some individuals may express concerns about meeting their nutritional needs, particularly in terms of protein intake.

However, this apprehension is largely unfounded. A well-planned plant-based diet can provide an abundance of protein from sources such as legumes, soy products, nuts, seeds, and even certain grains like quinoa. Additionally, the consumption of a variety of plant-based foods ensures a balanced intake of essential vitamins and minerals, mitigating the risk of nutrient deficiencies.

For those considering a transition to a plant-based lifestyle, gradual and sustainable changes are often recommended. Start by incorporating more plant-based meals into your weekly routine, experimenting with new recipes and flavor combinations. Explore different cuisines and cultures that have a rich tradition of plant-based cooking, such as Indian, Mediterranean, or Mexican cuisines. Seek guidance from healthcare professionals, nutritionists, or experienced plant-based advocates to ensure a smooth and well-informed transition.

Plant-based eating represents a holistic approach to nourishing the body, mind, and planet. By embracing the abundance of nature's offerings, individuals can unlock a myriad of health benefits, contribute to environmental sustainability, and align their dietary choices with ethical principles. Whether motivated by personal well-being, environmental concerns, or a desire for compassion towards all living beings, plant-based eating offers a path towards a more conscious and fulfilling way of life. Embark on this journey, one delicious and nourishing plant-based meal at a time, and experience the transformative power of nature's bounty.

Benefits of a plant-based diet for mental focus and energy

In the fast-paced, demanding world we live in, maintaining optimal mental focus and sustained energy levels is a constant challenge. From work deadlines to personal commitments, our cognitive abilities and physical vitality are put to the test daily. However, a growing body of research suggests that the key to unlocking our full mental and energetic potential may lie in the very foods we consume. Enter the plant-based diet, a dietary approach that harnesses the power of nature's bounty to enhance our cognitive performance and revitalize our energy reserves.

At its core, a plant-based diet emphasizes the consumption of whole, unprocessed foods derived from plants, including fruits, vegetables, whole grains, legumes, nuts, and seeds. By embracing this vibrant and nutrient-dense way of eating, individuals can experience a multitude of benefits that extend far beyond physical health, profoundly impacting their mental acuity and overall energy levels.

One of the primary advantages of a plant-based diet for mental focus is its ability to combat inflammation. Chronic inflammation has been linked to a range of cognitive impairments, including difficulties with memory, attention, and decision-making. Plant-based foods are rich in anti-inflammatory compounds, such as antioxidants, phytochemicals, and essential fatty acids, which work synergistically to reduce systemic inflammation and protect the brain from oxidative stress.

Antioxidants, abundant in fruits, vegetables, and many other plant-based foods, play a crucial role in neutralizing free radicals and mitigating the damage they can cause to brain cells. This protective mechanism helps maintain the integrity and optimal function of neurons, facilitating efficient communication and information processing within the brain.

Furthermore, plant-based diets are typically rich in fiber, a nutrient that has been shown to support cognitive function. Fiber not only promotes a healthy gut microbiome, which is increasingly recognized as having a profound impact on brain health, but it also helps regulate blood sugar levels. Stable blood sugar levels are essential for maintaining mental clarity and avoiding the cognitive fog and energy crashes associated with blood sugar spikes and dips.

Another key advantage of a plant-based diet for mental focus is its ability to improve blood flow and oxygen delivery to the brain. Many plant-based foods are rich in nitric oxide precursors, which help dilate blood vessels and increase circulation. This enhanced blood flow ensures that the brain receives an optimal supply of oxygen and nutrients, enabling it to function at its best.

Moreover, plant-based diets are often abundant in brain-boosting nutrients, such as omega-3 fatty acids, vitamin B12, folate, and choline. These essential nutrients play vital roles in neurotransmitter production, myelin formation (the insulation that surrounds nerve fibers), and overall brain health. By incorporating plant-based sources of these nutrients, such as walnuts, flaxseeds, fortified plant-based milks, and leafy greens, individuals can support their cognitive function and mental clarity.

Beyond the cognitive benefits, a plant-based diet can also provide a significant energy boost, combating fatigue and lethargy. Plant-based foods are typically lower in calories and higher in fiber, which can promote a healthy weight and prevent the sluggishness often associated with excess weight or poor digestion.

Additionally, the complex carbohydrates found in whole grains, legumes, and starchy vegetables provide a sustained release of energy, avoiding the energy crashes commonly experienced after consuming simple, refined carbohydrates. These nutrient-dense plant-based foods also supply an array of vitamins, minerals, and phytochemicals that support the body's energy production processes at the cellular level.

Furthermore, the alkaline nature of many plant-based foods can help counteract the acidic environment created by the consumption of animal products and processed foods. This alkaline state promotes optimal nutrient absorption and cellular function, contributing to increased energy levels and overall vitality.

For those concerned about meeting their protein needs on a plant-based diet, fear not. A well-planned, varied plant-based diet can provide ample amounts of high-quality protein from sources such as legumes, soy products, nuts, seeds, and even certain grains like quinoa. Adequate protein intake is essential for maintaining energy levels, as protein is involved in numerous metabolic processes and supports the growth and repair of tissues.

Transitioning to a plant-based diet can be a gradual and enjoyable process. Start by incorporating more plant-based meals into your weekly routine, experimenting with new recipes and flavor combinations. Seek guidance from healthcare professionals, nutritionists, or experienced plant-based advocates to ensure a balanced and nutrient-dense approach.

Embrace the vibrant colors, textures, and flavors of plant-based cuisine, and witness firsthand how this nourishing way of eating can transform your cognitive abilities and energy levels. From crisp salads bursting with nutrient-rich greens to hearty grain bowls adorned with roasted vegetables and plant-based proteins, the possibilities are endless.

In a world where mental focus and sustained energy are increasingly prized commodities, the plant-based diet emerges as a powerful ally. By harnessing the inherent power of nature's bounty, individuals can unlock their full cognitive potential, experience heightened mental clarity, and enjoy a revitalizing surge of energy. Embrace this transformative dietary approach and embark on a journey towards optimal mental performance and boundless vitality.

Overcoming common misconceptions about plant-based diets

In the realm of dietary choices, few topics have sparked as much debate and misconception as plant-based diets. From concerns about protein deficiencies to doubts regarding their ability to provide complete nutrition, these misconceptions have persisted, often overshadowing the numerous benefits that a well-planned plant-based lifestyle can offer. However, as scientific research continues to shed light on this subject, it becomes increasingly evident that many of these misconceptions are rooted in misinformation or outdated notions. In this part, we aim to dispel some of the most common myths surrounding plant-based diets, empowering individuals to make informed decisions about their dietary choices.

- **Myth #1: Plant-Based Diets Are Deficient in Protein**

One of the most prevalent misconceptions about plant-based diets is the belief that they are inherently lacking in protein, an essential macronutrient vital for various bodily functions, including muscle growth and repair, enzyme production, and hormone regulation. However, this notion is far from accurate. A well-planned plant-based diet can easily provide an adequate amount of high-quality protein from a variety of sources.

Legumes, such as lentils, chickpeas, and beans, are excellent sources of plant-based protein. For instance, a single cup of cooked lentils contains approximately 18 grams of protein. Soy products, including tofu, tempeh, and edamame, are also rich in protein, with tofu alone providing up to 20 grams of protein per cup. Nuts and seeds, like almonds, cashews, and chia seeds, are nutrient-dense and protein-packed additions to any plant-based diet.

Furthermore, many grains, such as quinoa, amaranth, and teff, are considered complete proteins, meaning they contain all nine essential amino acids required by the human body. By combining different plant-based protein sources in a meal or throughout the day, individuals can easily meet their protein requirements without relying on animal-based products.

- **Myth #2: Plant-Based Diets Lack Essential Nutrients**

Another common misconception surrounding plant-based diets is the belief that they are inherently lacking in essential nutrients, potentially leading to deficiencies. However, this notion is unfounded, as a well-planned and varied plant-based diet can provide all the necessary vitamins, minerals, and other vital nutrients required for optimal health.

Leafy green vegetables, such as spinach, kale, and collard greens, are rich sources of essential nutrients like iron, calcium, and vitamins A, C, and K. Whole grains, like brown rice, quinoa, and oats, provide a wealth of B vitamins, fiber, and essential minerals. Nuts and seeds are excellent sources of essential fatty acids, vitamins E and B6, and minerals like zinc and magnesium.

While some nutrients, such as vitamin B12, are primarily found in animal-based foods, many plant-based products are fortified with these essential nutrients. Additionally, individuals following a plant-based diet can supplement their diets with vitamin B12 or consume fortified plant-based milks, nutritional yeasts, or other fortified products to meet their needs.

- **Myth #3: Plant-Based Diets Are Boring and Restrictive**

Perhaps one of the most pervasive misconceptions about plant-based diets is the notion that they are inherently boring, restrictive, and lacking in variety. However, this belief could not be further from the truth. Plant-based cuisine encompasses a vast array of flavors, textures, and culinary traditions from around the globe, offering a diverse and exciting array of options for every palate.

From the vibrant and aromatic curries of Indian cuisine to the hearty and flavorful stews of the Mediterranean, plant-based cooking embraces a wealth of culinary traditions that have long celebrated the versatility and deliciousness of plant-based ingredients. The diversity of fruits, vegetables, grains, legumes, nuts, and seeds available provides an endless array of possibilities for creating delectable and satisfying meals.

Additionally, the rise of plant-based alternatives, such as meat substitutes, dairy-free cheeses, and egg replacements, has further expanded the culinary horizons of plant-based diets, allowing individuals to enjoy familiar flavors and textures while adhering to their dietary preferences.

- **Myth #4: Plant-Based Diets Are Expensive and Time-Consuming**

Another common misconception surrounding plant-based diets is the belief that they are inherently more expensive and time-consuming than traditional diets that include animal-based products. However, this assumption fails to consider the true cost and convenience of plant-based eating.

In reality, many plant-based staples, such as grains, legumes, and certain fruits and vegetables, are among the most affordable and accessible food items available. By focusing on simple, whole foods and minimizing the consumption of processed and packaged plant-based alternatives, individuals can enjoy a cost-effective and nutritious plant-based diet.

Furthermore, with the right planning and preparation techniques, plant-based meals can be just as convenient and time-efficient as any other dietary approach. Batch cooking, meal prepping, and embracing simple recipes that combine a few wholesome ingredients can streamline the cooking process and provide a steady supply of delicious, plant-based meals throughout the week.

- **Myth #5: Plant-Based Diets Are Unsuitable for Athletes and Active Individuals**

Lastly, a common misconception persists that plant-based diets are unsuitable for athletes and highly active individuals due to perceived limitations in protein and nutrient availability. However, this notion is contradicted by a growing body of evidence demonstrating that plant-based diets can not only meet the nutritional demands of active lifestyles but also offer potential performance advantages.

Many elite athletes and bodybuilders have successfully transitioned to plant-based diets, achieving impressive results in terms of strength, endurance, and recovery. Plant-based sources of protein, such as legumes, soy products, and grains, can provide high-quality, easily digestible protein to support muscle growth and repair.

Additionally, the anti-inflammatory properties of plant-based foods, coupled with their abundance of antioxidants and phytochemicals, can aid in recovery and reduce exercise-induced oxidative stress. The high-fiber content of plant-based diets may also contribute to improved gut health, which has been linked to better overall athletic performance and recovery.

By carefully planning their nutrient intake and ensuring adequate caloric consumption, plant-based athletes can not only meet their nutritional needs but also potentially experience performance benefits from this dietary approach.

While misconceptions surrounding plant-based diets persist, they are often rooted in misinformation or outdated beliefs. By separating fact from fiction and embracing the wealth of scientific evidence supporting the benefits of a well-planned plant-based lifestyle, individuals can make informed decisions about their dietary choices. Whether motivated by health concerns, environmental considerations, or ethical principles, a plant-based diet offers a nourishing and sustainable path to optimal well-being. It is time to shatter these myths and embrace the vibrant, nutrient-dense world of plant-based eating.

Setting the stage for success: kitchen essentials and pantry staples

Embarking on a plant-based dietary journey is an exciting and rewarding endeavor, offering a path to improved health, environmental sustainability, and ethical alignment. However, like any significant lifestyle change, proper preparation is key to ensuring long-term success. One of the most crucial steps in transitioning to a plant-based diet is creating a supportive environment within your own kitchen, stocking it with the essential tools and ingredients that will enable you to effortlessly prepare delicious, nutrient-dense meals.

In this part, we'll explore the essential kitchen equipment and pantry staples that will serve as the foundation for your plant-based culinary adventures. By equipping your kitchen with the right tools and stocking your pantry with versatile, nutrient-rich ingredients, you'll be well on your way to creating a seamless and enjoyable plant-based lifestyle.

- **Kitchen Essentials: Tools for Plant-Based Mastery**

➢ **High-Quality Knives:** Investing in a set of sharp, well-crafted knives is a must for any plant-based chef. From precisely slicing vegetables to breaking down sturdy produce like squash or pineapples, a good set of knives will make food preparation a breeze and ensure efficiency in the kitchen.

➤ **Versatile Cookware:** A non-stick skillet, a heavy-bottomed pot for simmering soups and stews, and a baking sheet for roasting vegetables are essential components of a plant-based kitchen. Consider investing in high-quality, durable cookware that will stand the test of time and make meal preparation a joy.

➤ **Blender or Food Processor:** A powerful blender or food processor is an invaluable asset in the plant-based kitchen. From whipping up creamy smoothies and nut butters to creating velvety soups and dips, these versatile appliances will become your go-to tools for effortless meal prep.

➢ **Spiralizer or Vegetable Peeler:** For those seeking creative ways to incorporate more vegetables into their diet, a spiralizer or julienne peeler can transform ordinary produce into fun, noodle-like strands or ribbons, adding variety and visual appeal to your plant-based dishes.

➢ **Nut Milk Bag or Cheesecloth:** For those interested in making their own plant-based milks or straining broths and sauces, a nut milk bag or cheesecloth is an indispensable item. These simple tools allow you to easily separate liquids from solids, ensuring smooth and creamy textures in your culinary creations.

- **Pantry Staples: Building Blocks of Plant-Based Nutrition**

➢ **Whole Grains:** Whole grains like quinoa, brown rice, farro, and whole-wheat pasta should be staples in any plant-based pantry. Not only are they excellent sources of complex carbohydrates and fiber, but they also provide a versatile base for countless meals and can be easily dressed up with an array of vegetables, legumes, and flavorful sauces.

➢ **Legumes:** Lentils, chickpeas, black beans, and kidney beans are nutritional powerhouses that should have a permanent place in your pantry. These protein-packed, fiber-rich foods can be incorporated into various dishes, from hearty soups and stews to flavorful curries and veggie burgers.

➢ **Nuts and Seeds:** Almonds, cashews, walnuts, pumpkin seeds, and chia seeds are excellent sources of healthy fats, plant-based protein, and a wide range of essential nutrients. They can be used as toppings, incorporated into baked goods, or transformed into delicious nut butters and milks.

➢ **Dried Fruits and Vegetables:** Keeping a selection of dried fruits like raisins, apricots, and cranberries, as well as dried vegetables like sun-dried tomatoes and mushrooms, can add depth of flavor and texture to your plant-based meals. They also make for convenient, nutrient-dense snacks on the go.

➢ **Herbs and Spices:** A well-stocked spice rack is the key to elevating the flavors of your plant-based dishes. Invest in a variety of dried herbs, spices, and spice blends to add depth, complexity, and cultural flair to your culinary creations.

➢ **Plant-Based Milks and Alternatives:** From soy milk and almond milk to coconut yogurt and vegan cheese alternatives, these plant-based substitutes can help recreate familiar flavors and textures while adhering to your dietary preferences.

➢ **Condiments and Sauces:** Stock your pantry with a variety of plant-based condiments and sauces, such as tamari or soy sauce, tahini, nut butters, vinegars, and hot sauces. These versatile additions can transform simple dishes into flavor-packed masterpieces.

➢ **Vegetable and Fruit Staples:** While fresh produce should be a priority, it's also helpful to keep a selection of canned or frozen fruits and vegetables on hand. These shelf-stable options can be convenient backups when fresh produce is scarce, ensuring that you always have access to nutritious plant-based ingredients.

● **Creating a Supportive Kitchen Environment**

Beyond stocking your kitchen with the right tools and ingredients, there are a few additional steps you can take to create an environment that supports and encourages your plant-based lifestyle:

- ➢ **Meal Planning and Preparation:** Dedicating time each week to plan your meals and prepare ingredients in advance can make plant-based cooking a breeze. Batch cooking grains, roasting vegetables, and portioning out ingredients for the week ahead can save you valuable time and ensure that you always have nourishing options at your fingertips.

- ➢ **Recipe Resources:** Invest in a few high-quality plant-based cookbooks or bookmark reliable online recipe sources. These resources will provide you with a wealth of inspiration and guidance, helping you explore new flavors and techniques while expanding your plant-based repertoire.

➢ **Community Support:** Connecting with like-minded individuals can be a powerful motivator on your plant-based journey. Join online forums, local meetup groups, or attend plant-based cooking classes to share tips, recipes, and encouragement with others who share your dietary values.

➢ **Mindset Shift:** Embrace the plant-based lifestyle as an opportunity for culinary exploration and personal growth. Rather than viewing it as a restriction, approach it as a chance to discover new flavors, cooking techniques, and cultural traditions while nourishing your body and aligning with your values.

By thoughtfully stocking your kitchen with the right tools and pantry staples, and creating a supportive environment that fosters your plant-based journey, you'll be setting the stage for long-term success. With a well-equipped kitchen and a pantry brimming with nutrient-rich ingredients, the possibilities for delicious, satisfying, and health-promoting plant-based meals are truly endless.

Embrace this exciting culinary journey, savor each flavorful creation, and revel in the knowledge that you are nourishing your body, respecting the environment, and aligning your choices with your ethical principles. Welcome to the vibrant and nourishing world of plant-based living!

Chapter 2

Understanding Nutritional Needs

Essential nutrients in a plant-based diet

Embracing a plant-based diet has gained significant traction in recent years, driven by concerns for personal health, environmental sustainability, and ethical considerations. While this dietary approach offers numerous benefits, ensuring adequate intake of essential nutrients is crucial for maintaining overall well-being. In this comprehensive discussion, we will explore the key nutrients found in plant-based diets and provide practical strategies for achieving a balanced and nutritious lifestyle.

➢ **Protein:** Contrary to popular belief, plant-based diets can provide ample protein from a variety of sources. Legumes, such as lentils, chickpeas, and beans, are excellent sources of protein, offering a range of amino acids essential for tissue repair, enzyme production, and immune function. Nuts and seeds, including almonds, chia seeds, and hemp seeds, are also rich in protein and beneficial fats. Additionally, whole grains like quinoa and amaranth are considered complete protein sources, containing all nine essential amino acids.

➤ **Omega-3 Fatty Acids:** Omega-3 fatty acids are essential for maintaining cardiovascular health, brain function, and reducing inflammation. While plant-based diets lack the readily available omega-3s found in fatty fish, there are alternative sources. Flaxseeds, chia seeds, walnuts, and hemp seeds are excellent sources of alpha-linolenic acid (ALA), a precursor to the more bioavailable forms of omega-3s. Additionally, algae-based supplements can provide direct sources of EPA and DHA, the most biologically active forms of omega-3s.

➤ **Iron:** Iron is a crucial mineral for oxygen transport and energy production. Plant-based sources of iron include fortified cereals, legumes, nuts, seeds, and dark leafy greens like spinach and Swiss chard. However, the iron in plant-based foods is less bioavailable than that found in animal products. To enhance iron absorption, it is recommended to pair iron-rich foods with vitamin C-rich sources, such as bell peppers, citrus fruits, and tomatoes.

➢ **Calcium:** Calcium is essential for maintaining strong bones and teeth, as well as supporting muscle function and nerve transmission. While dairy products are often associated with calcium, plant-based sources like tofu, tempeh, leafy greens, fortified plant-based milks, and calcium-set tofu can provide adequate amounts of this vital mineral. Additionally, consuming foods rich in vitamin D, such as mushrooms and fortified plant-based milks, can enhance calcium absorption.

➢ **Vitamin B12:** Vitamin B12 is crucial for red blood cell formation, neurological function, and DNA synthesis. Since this vitamin is primarily found in animal products, individuals following a strict plant-based diet may be at risk of deficiency. Fortified plant-based milks, nutritional yeast, and some meat substitutes can provide a reliable source of vitamin B12. Alternatively, supplementation may be necessary for those with limited access to fortified foods.

➢ **Zinc:** Zinc plays a vital role in immune function, wound healing, and protein synthesis. Plant-based sources of zinc include whole grains, legumes, nuts, and seeds. However, the bioavailability of zinc from plant-based sources can be hindered by the presence of phytates, compounds found in grains and legumes that bind to minerals. Soaking, sprouting, and fermenting these foods can help reduce phytate levels and improve zinc absorption.

To ensure a well-rounded and nutrient-dense plant-based diet, it is essential to incorporate a diverse array of whole, minimally processed foods. This includes a variety of fruits, vegetables, whole grains, legumes, nuts, and seeds. Additionally, fortified plant-based milks, nutritional yeast, and meat substitutes can provide supplementary sources of essential nutrients.

Meal planning and preparation techniques can further enhance the nutritional value of plant-based dishes. For example, soaking and sprouting nuts, seeds, and legumes can increase nutrient bioavailability, while combining complementary protein sources, such as rice and beans, can provide a complete array of essential amino acids.

It is also crucial to address potential nutrient gaps through careful planning or supplementation, as individual needs may vary based on age, gender, activity level, and specific health conditions. Consulting with a qualified healthcare professional or registered dietitian can help ensure that your plant-based diet meets your unique nutritional requirements.

A well-planned and diverse plant-based diet can provide an abundance of essential nutrients necessary for optimal health and well-being. By embracing a variety of whole, minimally processed plant-based foods, incorporating nutrient-dense ingredients, and employing appropriate cooking techniques, individuals can enjoy the numerous benefits of this dietary approach while meeting their nutritional needs. Embracing a plant-based lifestyle not only contributes to personal well-being but also promotes environmental sustainability and aligns with ethical values, making it a choice that resonates with multiple aspects of a conscious and fulfilling life.

How to ensure you're getting enough protein, iron, calcium, etc.

Transitioning to a plant-based diet can be a rewarding journey, offering numerous health benefits, environmental advantages, and ethical considerations. However, one of the common concerns voiced by those contemplating or following this dietary approach is the potential for nutrient deficiencies, particularly when it comes to essential nutrients like protein, iron, calcium, and others. In this comprehensive guide, we'll explore practical strategies to ensure you're meeting your nutritional needs while embracing a plant-based lifestyle.

- **Protein: Building Blocks for Vitality**

Protein is a macronutrient that plays a crucial role in various bodily functions, including tissue repair, enzyme production, and immune function. While many associate protein primarily with animal sources, plant-based diets can provide ample protein from a variety of whole, minimally processed foods.

a. Legumes: Lentils, chickpeas, black beans, and kidney beans are excellent sources of plant-based protein, offering a range of amino acids essential for overall health.

b. Nuts and Seeds: Almonds, cashews, pumpkin seeds, and chia seeds are not only rich in protein but also provide beneficial fats and fiber.

c. Whole Grains: Quinoa, amaranth, and brown rice are considered complete protein sources, containing all nine essential amino acids.

d. Soy Products: Tempeh, tofu, and edamame are versatile soy-based protein sources that can be incorporated into various dishes.

To ensure optimal protein intake, consider combining different plant-based protein sources in a single meal or throughout the day. This practice, known as "protein combining," helps provide a complete amino acid profile.

- **Iron: Fueling Oxygen Transport**

Iron is a vital mineral responsible for oxygen transport and energy production. While plant-based diets can provide sufficient iron, it's important to note that the iron found in plant sources (non-heme iron) is less bioavailable than the heme iron found in animal products.

a. Lentils, spinach, cashews, and quinoa are excellent sources of plant-based iron.

b. Enhance iron absorption by pairing iron-rich foods with vitamin C-rich sources like bell peppers, citrus fruits, and tomatoes.

c. Consider cooking in cast-iron cookware, as a small amount of iron can leach into the food during the cooking process.

d. Avoid consuming iron-rich foods with calcium-rich foods or beverages, as calcium can inhibit iron absorption.

- **Calcium: Building Strong Bones and Teeth**

Calcium is essential for maintaining strong bones and teeth, as well as supporting muscle function and nerve transmission. While dairy products are often associated with calcium, plant-based diets offer a variety of calcium-rich options.

a. Leafy greens like kale, collard greens, and bok choy are excellent sources of calcium.

b. Fortified plant-based milks, such as soy, almond, and oat milk, can provide significant amounts of calcium.

c. Tofu, tempeh, and calcium-set tofu are soy-based sources of calcium.

d. Incorporate sesame seeds, tahini (sesame seed paste), and almonds into your diet for additional calcium.

To enhance calcium absorption, ensure adequate vitamin D intake from sources like fortified plant-based milks, mushrooms exposed to UV light, or a supplement if necessary.

- **Omega-3 Fatty Acids: Promoting Heart and Brain Health**

Omega-3 fatty acids are essential for maintaining cardiovascular health, brain function, and reducing inflammation. While plant-based diets lack the readily available omega-3s found in fatty fish, there are alternative sources to consider.

a. Flaxseeds, chia seeds, walnuts, and hemp seeds are excellent sources of alpha-linolenic acid (ALA), a precursor to the more bioavailable forms of omega-3s.

b. Incorporate algae-based supplements, which can provide direct sources of EPA and DHA, the most biologically active forms of omega-3s.

c. Consider fortified plant-based milks, juices, and other products enriched with omega-3s from microalgae sources.

- **Vitamin B12: Supporting Red Blood Cell Formation and Neurological Function**

Vitamin B12 is crucial for red blood cell formation, neurological function, and DNA synthesis. Since this vitamin is primarily found in animal products, individuals following a strict plant-based diet may be at risk of deficiency.

a. Fortified plant-based milks, nutritional yeast, and some meat substitutes can provide reliable sources of vitamin B12.

b. Supplementation with a high-quality vitamin B12 supplement may be necessary, especially for those with limited access to fortified foods.

c. Consult with a healthcare professional or registered dietitian to determine the appropriate dose and form of vitamin B12 supplementation based on your individual needs.

- **Zinc: Supporting Immune Function and Wound Healing**

Zinc plays a vital role in immune function, wound healing, and protein synthesis. While plant-based sources can provide zinc, the bioavailability of this mineral can be hindered by the presence of phytates, compounds found in grains and legumes that bind to minerals.

a. Whole grains, legumes, nuts, and seeds are good sources of plant-based zinc.

b. Soaking, sprouting, and fermenting grains and legumes can help reduce phytate levels and improve zinc absorption.

c. Combine zinc-rich foods with vitamin C-rich sources, as vitamin C can enhance zinc absorption.

d. Consider supplementation with a high-quality zinc supplement if deemed necessary by a healthcare professional.

- **Meal Planning and Preparation Techniques**

To optimize nutrient intake and ensure a well-rounded plant-based diet, incorporate the following meal planning and preparation techniques:

a. Embrace a diverse array of whole, minimally processed plant-based foods, including fruits, vegetables, whole grains, legumes, nuts, and seeds.

b. Combine complementary protein sources, such as rice and beans or whole-wheat bread and hummus, to provide a complete amino acid profile.

c. Soak, sprout, and ferment grains, legumes, nuts, and seeds to enhance nutrient bioavailability and reduce anti-nutrient content.

d. Incorporate nutrient-dense ingredients like nutritional yeast, sea vegetables, and fortified plant-based products to boost micronutrient intake.

e. Consult with a qualified healthcare professional or registered dietitian, especially if you have specific health concerns or dietary restrictions, to ensure your plant-based diet meets your unique nutritional needs.

Transitioning to a plant-based diet requires mindful planning and education to ensure you're meeting your body's nutrient requirements. By incorporating a variety of whole, minimally processed plant-based foods, employing appropriate preparation techniques, and embracing nutrient-dense ingredients, you can enjoy the numerous benefits of this dietary approach while maintaining optimal health and well-being.

Remember, a well-planned and diverse plant-based diet can provide an abundance of essential nutrients, promoting vitality, longevity, and overall wellness. Embrace this lifestyle with confidence, and experience the transformative power of nourishing your body with nature's bounty.

Balancing macronutrients for sustained energy

Embracing a plant-based diet offers a myriad of benefits for both personal well-being and environmental sustainability. However, one crucial aspect that often raises concerns is the ability to maintain sustained energy levels throughout the day. Balancing macronutrients

– carbohydrates, proteins, and fats – is key to ensuring you have the fuel your body needs to perform optimally, whether you're tackling daily tasks, engaging in physical activities, or simply striving for overall vitality. In this comprehensive guide, we'll explore practical strategies to achieve a well-balanced macronutrient profile within a plant-based dietary approach.

- **Carbohydrates: The Body's Primary Fuel Source**

Carbohydrates are the body's primary source of energy, providing the glucose necessary for powering various bodily functions, including brain activity and muscle contractions. When it comes to plant-based diets, carbohydrates can be obtained from a variety of nutrient-dense sources.

a. Whole Grains: Opt for whole, minimally processed grains like quinoa, brown rice, oats, and whole-wheat bread or pasta. These complex carbohydrates provide a steady supply of energy, fiber, and essential nutrients.

b. Fruits and Vegetables: Load up on a rainbow of fruits and vegetables, which offer not only carbohydrates but also a wealth of vitamins, minerals, antioxidants, and fiber.

c. Legumes: Lentils, chickpeas, black beans, and other legumes are excellent sources of complex carbohydrates, providing sustained energy and beneficial fiber.

d. Tubers: Sweet potatoes, potatoes, and other starchy vegetables can serve as a reliable source of carbohydrates and micronutrients.

To maintain consistent energy levels throughout the day, it's essential to incorporate a balanced combination of complex carbohydrates and fiber-rich foods into your meals and snacks. This approach helps regulate blood sugar levels and prevents energy crashes.

- **Protein: Building Blocks for Sustained Vitality**

Protein plays a crucial role in numerous bodily functions, including tissue repair, enzyme production, and immune support. While many associate protein primarily with animal sources, plant-based diets offer a wide array of protein-rich options to fuel your body and maintain energy levels.

a. Legumes: Lentils, chickpeas, black beans, and other legumes are not only excellent sources of complex carbohydrates but also provide a generous amount of plant-based protein.

b. Soy Products: Tempeh, tofu, and edamame are versatile soy-based protein sources that can be incorporated into a variety of dishes.

c. Nuts and Seeds: Almonds, cashews, pumpkin seeds, and chia seeds are nutrient-dense snacks that offer both protein and healthy fats.

d. Whole Grains: Quinoa, amaranth, and buckwheat are considered complete protein sources, containing all nine essential amino acids.

To ensure optimal protein intake and sustained energy levels, consider combining different plant-based protein sources in a single meal or throughout the day. This practice, known as "protein combining," helps provide a complete amino acid profile.

- **Fats: Fueling Energy and Supporting Nutrient Absorption**

While often vilified, fats are an essential macronutrient that plays a crucial role in energy production, nutrient absorption, and overall health. When it comes to plant-based diets, it's important to focus on healthy, unsaturated fats.

a. Nuts and Seeds: Almonds, walnuts, chia seeds, and flaxseeds are excellent sources of heart-healthy unsaturated fats, providing lasting energy and satiety.

b. Avocados: Rich in monounsaturated fats, avocados are a nutrient-dense addition to any plant-based diet, offering a creamy texture and versatility in various dishes.

c. Olive Oil and Coconut Oil: These plant-based oils can be used for cooking and dressing, providing a source of healthy fats and enhancing the absorption of fat-soluble vitamins.

d. Nut and Seed Butters: Almond butter, peanut butter, and tahini (sesame seed paste) offer a convenient way to incorporate healthy fats into your diet, while also providing protein and fiber.

Incorporating adequate amounts of healthy fats into your plant-based diet not only supports sustained energy levels but also aids in nutrient absorption and promotes overall satiety, reducing the risk of overeating or energy crashes.

- **Meal Planning and Preparation Techniques**

To ensure a well-balanced macronutrient profile and sustained energy levels throughout the day, consider implementing the following meal planning and preparation techniques:

a. Embrace a variety of whole, minimally processed plant-based foods, including fruits, vegetables, whole grains, legumes, nuts, and seeds.

b. Plan your meals and snacks to include a combination of complex carbohydrates, plant-based proteins, and healthy fats to promote lasting energy and satiety.

c. Experiment with plant-based protein sources like tempeh, seitan, and meat substitutes to add variety and ensure adequate protein intake.

d. Incorporate nutrient-dense ingredients like chia seeds, flaxseeds, and hemp seeds to boost your intake of healthy fats and plant-based proteins.

e. Stay hydrated by drinking plenty of water and incorporating hydrating fruits and vegetables into your diet, as proper hydration is essential for optimal energy levels.

f. Consider consulting with a qualified healthcare professional or registered dietitian, especially if you have specific health concerns or dietary restrictions, to ensure your plant-based diet meets your unique nutritional needs and energy requirements.

- **Mindful Eating and Listening to Your Body's Cues**

In addition to carefully planning your meals and snacks, it's essential to cultivate mindful eating habits and tune into your body's cues. By doing so, you can better understand your energy levels and adjust your macronutrient intake accordingly.

a. Practice portion control and pay attention to hunger and fullness cues to prevent overeating or undereating.

b. Observe how different foods and macronutrient ratios affect your energy levels, and make adjustments as needed.

c. Engage in regular physical activity, as exercise not only supports energy expenditure but also can improve nutrient utilization and overall well-being.

d. Prioritize quality sleep, as adequate rest is crucial for optimal energy levels and overall health.

By embracing a well-balanced plant-based diet rich in complex carbohydrates, plant-based proteins, and healthy fats, you can experience sustained energy levels throughout the day. Remember, every individual has unique nutritional needs and preferences, so it's essential to experiment and find the macronutrient balance that works best for your lifestyle and personal goals.

Balancing macronutrients within a plant-based dietary approach is not only achievable but also incredibly rewarding. By nourishing your body with a diverse array of whole, nutrient-dense plant foods, you'll experience a newfound sense of vitality and energy, fueling your passion for life and enabling you to tackle each day with vigor and enthusiasm.

Tips for meal planning and prepping to meet your nutritional needs

Proper meal planning and preparation are essential to achieving a well-balanced, nutrient-dense diet that supports optimal health and vitality. In this comprehensive guide, we'll explore practical tips and strategies to help you streamline your meal planning and prepping efforts, enabling you to thrive on a plant-based diet.

- **Assess Your Nutritional Needs**

  Before diving into meal planning and prepping, it's crucial to understand your unique nutritional requirements. Consider factors such as age, gender, activity level, and any specific health concerns or dietary restrictions. This information will serve as the foundation for creating a tailored meal plan that meets your individual needs.

a. Consult with a qualified healthcare professional or registered dietitian, especially if you have specific medical conditions or dietary restrictions, to ensure your plant-based diet meets your unique nutritional needs.

b. Utilize online nutrient calculators or tracking apps to estimate your daily caloric and macronutrient (protein, carbohydrates, and fats) requirements, as well as recommended intakes for essential vitamins and minerals.

c. Familiarize yourself with nutrient-dense plant-based foods that can help you meet your nutritional goals, such as legumes, nuts, seeds, whole grains, and a variety of fruits and vegetables.

- **Embrace Meal Planning**

Effective meal planning is the key to ensuring you have a steady supply of nutritious, plant-based meals and snacks readily available. This practice not only saves time and reduces stress but also helps you stay on track with your dietary goals.

a. Start by creating a weekly or monthly meal plan that incorporates a variety of plant-based foods, including protein sources, complex carbohydrates, healthy fats, and an abundance of fruits and vegetables.

b. Consider batch cooking or meal prepping on weekends or designated days to have ready-to-eat meals and snacks on hand for busy weekdays.

c. Utilize online resources, plant-based cookbooks, or meal planning apps to find inspiring recipes and meal ideas that align with your dietary preferences and nutritional needs.

d. Plan for variety and incorporate different cuisines, flavors, and cooking techniques to prevent boredom and ensure you're getting a diverse range of nutrients.

- **Stock Your Pantry and Fridge**

Having a well-stocked pantry and refrigerator with plant-based staples and fresh produce will make meal planning and prepping more accessible and efficient.

a. Stock your pantry with shelf-stable items like whole grains (quinoa, brown rice, oats), legumes (lentils, chickpeas, black beans), nuts and seeds, nut butters, and plant-based milks.

b. Keep your refrigerator stocked with fresh fruits and vegetables, tofu, tempeh, plant-based protein sources, and condiments like hummus or tahini.

c. Invest in airtight containers, reusable bags, and meal prep containers to store prepped ingredients, meals, and snacks, ensuring they stay fresh and organized.

d. Take advantage of seasonal produce and bulk-buying options to save money and reduce food waste.

- **Batch Cooking and Meal Prepping Strategies**

Batch cooking and meal prepping are game-changers when it comes to maintaining a plant-based diet. These strategies not only save time but also ensure you have a steady supply of nutritious meals and snacks readily available.

a. Dedicate a specific day or block of time each week for batch cooking and meal prepping.

b. Cook larger portions of staple items like grains, legumes, and roasted vegetables, which can be easily repurposed into multiple meals throughout the week.

c. Prepare and portion out individual components like marinated tofu, roasted potatoes, or quinoa salad, which can be combined in various ways for quick and easy meal assembly.

d. Consider freezing portions of soups, stews, or casseroles for future use, ensuring you have nutritious options on hand for busy days.

- **Simplify with Plant-Based Meal Delivery Services**

If meal planning and prepping feel overwhelming, consider exploring plant-based meal delivery services. These services can provide a convenient and hassle-free way to ensure you're meeting your nutritional needs while adhering to a plant-based diet.

a. Research and compare different plant-based meal delivery services to find one that aligns with your dietary preferences, budget, and nutritional requirements.

b. Look for services that offer a variety of meal options, use high-quality ingredients, and provide detailed nutritional information.

c. Meal delivery services can be especially helpful for those with hectic schedules, limited cooking skills, or specific dietary restrictions.

d. Supplement the delivered meals with fresh fruits, vegetables, and other plant-based snacks to ensure a well-rounded diet.

- **Embrace Mindful Eating and Portion Control**

While meal planning and prepping are essential, it's equally important to cultivate mindful eating habits and practice portion control to support your nutritional goals.

a. Tune into your body's hunger and fullness cues to avoid overeating or undereating.

b. Practice mindful eating by savoring each bite, chewing thoroughly, and acknowledging the flavors and textures of your food.

c. Use smaller plates or bowls to control portion sizes and prevent overeating.

d. Stay hydrated by drinking plenty of water throughout the day, as proper hydration supports overall health and can aid in regulating appetite.

- **Involve Family and Friends**

Meal planning and prepping can be more enjoyable and sustainable when you involve family members or friends. Embracing a plant-based lifestyle as a collective effort can foster accountability, shared knowledge, and a sense of community.

a. Involve family members or friends in the meal planning process, encouraging them to share their favorite plant-based recipes and meal ideas.

b. Host potluck-style gatherings where everyone contributes a plant-based dish, allowing you to sample a variety of flavors and expand your culinary repertoire.

c. Engage children in age-appropriate meal prepping tasks, such as washing produce or assembling simple snacks, to foster healthy eating habits from an early age.

d. Share your plant-based meal planning and prepping tips with others, inspiring and supporting those interested in adopting a more sustainable and nutritious lifestyle.

By implementing these practical tips and strategies, meal planning and prepping for a plant-based diet becomes a seamless and rewarding experience. Not only will you ensure you're meeting your nutritional needs, but you'll also save time, reduce stress, and cultivate a healthier relationship with food. Embrace this journey with enthusiasm and an open mind, and you'll soon discover the abundance of flavors, textures, and nourishment that a well-planned, plant-based diet has to offer.

Chapter 3

Breakfast Boosters

Avocado Toast

Description: A simple yet delicious breakfast or snack option featuring creamy avocado spread on toasted bread.

Preparation time: 5 minutes

Cooking time: 5 minutes

Number of servings: 2

Ingredients:

- 2 ripe avocados

- 4 slices of whole grain bread

- Salt and pepper to taste

- Optional toppings: cherry tomatoes, red pepper flakes, sesame seeds, or a drizzle of balsamic glaze

Instructions:

1. Slice the avocados in half and remove the pits. Scoop out the flesh into a bowl and mash it with a fork until smooth.

2. Toast the bread slices until golden brown and crispy.

3. Spread the mashed avocado evenly onto the toasted bread slices.

4. Season with salt and pepper to taste.

5. Garnish with your choice of optional toppings,
    if desired.

    Nutritional info: (Per serving)

- Calories: 250

- Fat: 15g

- Carbohydrates: 25g

- Protein: 5g

Smoothie Bowl

Description: A refreshing and nutritious breakfast or snack option packed with fruits, veggies, and your favorite toppings.

Preparation time: 10 minutes

Number of servings: 2

Ingredients:

- 2 ripe bananas, frozen

- 1 cup mixed berries (strawberries, blueberries, raspberries)

- 1 cup spinach leaves

- 1/2 cup almond milk (or any plant-based milk)

- Toppings: granola, sliced fruits, shredded coconut, chia seeds, or nuts

Instructions:

1. In a blender, combine the frozen bananas, mixed berries, spinach, and almond milk.

2. Blend until smooth and creamy, adding more almond milk if needed to reach your desired consistency.

3. Pour the smoothie into bowls.

4. Top with your favorite toppings such as granola, sliced fruits, shredded coconut, chia seeds, or nuts.

5. Serve immediately and enjoy!

Nutritional info: (Per serving)

- Calories: 200

- Fat: 5g

- Carbohydrates: 40g

- Protein: 4g

Chia Pudding

Description: A healthy and satisfying dessert or breakfast option made with chia seeds soaked in creamy coconut milk.

Preparation time: 5 minutes (plus chilling time)

Number of servings: 2

Ingredients:

- 1/4 cup chia seeds

- 1 cup coconut milk (or any plant-based milk)

- 1 tablespoon maple syrup (or sweetener of choice)

- 1/2 teaspoon vanilla extract

- Fresh fruit or berries for topping

Instructions:

1. In a bowl, whisk together the chia seeds, coconut milk, maple syrup, and vanilla extract until well combined.

2. Cover the bowl and refrigerate for at least 2 hours or overnight, allowing the chia seeds to absorb the liquid and thicken.

3. Stir the chia pudding mixture before serving to ensure it's well mixed.

4. Divide the chia pudding into serving bowls.

5. Top with fresh fruit or berries before serving.

6. Enjoy chilled!

Nutritional info: (Per serving)

- Calories: 180

- Fat: 12g

- Carbohydrates: 15g

- Protein: 4g

Vegan Pancakes

Description: Fluffy and delicious pancakes made without eggs or dairy, perfect for a weekend breakfast treat.

Preparation time: 10 minutes

Cooking time: 10 minutes

Number of servings: 4

Ingredients:

- 1 cup all-purpose flour

- 1 tablespoon sugar

- 2 teaspoons baking powder

- 1/4 teaspoon salt

- 1 cup almond milk (or any plant-based milk)

- 2 tablespoons coconut oil (melted)

- 1 teaspoon vanilla extract

Instructions:

1. In a large mixing bowl, whisk together the flour, sugar, baking powder, and salt.

2. In a separate bowl, mix together the almond milk, melted coconut oil, and vanilla extract.

3. Pour the wet ingredients into the dry ingredients and stir until just combined. Do not overmix; lumps are okay.

4. Heat a non-stick skillet or griddle over medium heat and lightly grease with coconut oil or cooking spray.

5. Pour about 1/4 cup of batter onto the skillet for each pancake.

6. Cook until bubbles form on the surface of the pancake, then flip and cook until golden brown on the other side.

7. Repeat with the remaining batter.

8. Serve warm with your favorite toppings such as maple syrup, fresh fruit, or vegan butter.

Nutritional info: (Per serving, without toppings)

- Calories: 180

- Fat: 7g

- Carbohydrates: 25g

- Protein: 3g

Tofu Scramble

Description: A satisfying and protein-packed alternative to scrambled eggs, made with tofu and flavorful spices.

Preparation time: 10 minutes

Cooking time: 10 minutes

Number of servings: 2

Ingredients:

- 1 block firm tofu, drained and pressed

- 1 tablespoon olive oil

- 1/2 onion, diced

- 1 bell pepper, diced

- 2 cloves garlic, minced

- 1 teaspoon turmeric

- 1/2 teaspoon cumin

- 1/2 teaspoon paprika

- Salt and pepper to taste

- Optional add-ins: spinach, mushrooms, tomatoes, nutritional yeast

Instructions:

1. Crumble the pressed tofu into a bowl using your hands or a fork.

2. Heat the olive oil in a skillet over medium heat.

3. Add the diced onion and bell pepper to the skillet and sauté until softened, about 3-4 minutes.

4. Add the minced garlic to the skillet and cook for another 1-2 minutes until fragrant.

5. Stir in the crumbled tofu, turmeric, cumin, paprika, salt, and pepper. Mix well to combine.

6. Cook for 5-7 minutes, stirring occasionally, until the tofu is heated through and slightly browned.

7. If using any optional add-ins, add them to the skillet and cook until heated through.

8. Adjust seasoning to taste and serve hot.

Nutritional info: (Per serving)

- Calories: 200

- Fat: 12g

- Carbohydrates: 8g

- Protein: 15g

Overnight Oats

Description: A convenient and nutritious breakfast option made by soaking oats overnight with your choice of milk and toppings.

Preparation time: 5 minutes (plus overnight soaking)

Number of servings: 2

Ingredients:

- 1 cup rolled oats
- 1 cup almond milk (or any plant-based milk)
- 2 tablespoons chia seeds
- 1 tablespoon maple syrup (or sweetener of choice)
- 1/2 teaspoon vanilla extract
- Toppings: sliced fruits, nuts, seeds, or nut butter

Instructions:

1. In a bowl or jar, combine the rolled oats, almond milk, chia seeds, maple syrup, and vanilla extract.

2. Stir well to combine all ingredients.

3. Cover the bowl or jar and refrigerate overnight, or for at least 4 hours, to allow the oats to soften and absorb the liquid.

4. In the morning, give the oats a good stir and add more milk if desired to reach your preferred consistency.

5. Top with sliced fruits, nuts, seeds, or a dollop of nut butter before serving.

6. Enjoy cold or gently warmed!

Nutritional info: (Per serving)

- Calories: 250

- Fat: 8g

- Carbohydrates: 40g

- Protein: 7g

Fruit Salad

Description: A refreshing and colorful combination of fresh fruits tossed together for a light and healthy breakfast or snack.

Preparation time: 10 minutes

Number of servings: 4

Ingredients:

- 2 apples, diced

- 2 bananas, sliced

- 1 cup strawberries, hulled and halved

- 1 cup grapes, halved

- 1 cup pineapple chunks

- Juice of 1 lemon

- Optional: honey or maple syrup for drizzling

Instructions:

1. In a large bowl, combine all the diced and sliced fruits.

2. Squeeze the lemon juice over the fruits and gently toss to coat, to prevent them from browning.

3. Drizzle with honey or maple syrup if desired, for added sweetness.

4. Serve immediately or refrigerate until ready to serve.

5. Enjoy this vibrant and flavorful fruit salad!

Nutritional info: (Per serving)

- Calories: 120

- Fat: 0.5g

- Carbohydrates: 30g

- Protein: 1g

Veggie Breakfast Burrito

Description: A hearty and satisfying breakfast option filled with scrambled tofu, sautéed vegetables, and flavorful spices, wrapped in a warm tortilla.

Preparation time: 15 minutes

Cooking time: 15 minutes

Number of servings: 2

Ingredients:

- 1 block firm tofu, drained and pressed

- 1 tablespoon olive oil

- 1/2 onion, diced

- 1 bell pepper, diced

- 1 cup spinach leaves

- 1 teaspoon turmeric

- 1/2 teaspoon cumin

- Salt and pepper to taste

- 2 large tortillas (whole wheat or gluten-free)

- Optional toppings: salsa, avocado, vegan cheese

Instructions:

1. Crumble the pressed tofu into a bowl using your hands or a fork.

2. Heat the olive oil in a skillet over medium heat.

3. Add the diced onion and bell pepper to the
    skillet and sauté until softened, about 3-4
    minutes.

4. Add the spinach leaves to the skillet and cook
    until wilted, about 1-2 minutes.

5. Stir in the crumbled tofu, turmeric, cumin, salt,
    and pepper. Mix well to combine.

6. Cook for 5-7 minutes, stirring occasionally,
    until the tofu is heated through and slightly
    browned.

7. Warm the tortillas in a separate skillet or
    microwave.

8. Divide the tofu mixture evenly between the
    tortillas.

9. Add any optional toppings such as salsa,
    avocado, or vegan cheese.

10. Roll up the tortillas tightly to form burritos.

11. Serve immediately, or wrap in foil to take on

the go!

Nutritional info: (Per serving)

- Calories: 300

- Fat: 12g

- Carbohydrates: 25g

- Protein: 15g

Quinoa Breakfast Bowl

Description: A nutritious and filling breakfast option featuring fluffy quinoa topped with fresh fruits, nuts, and a drizzle of maple syrup.

Preparation time: 15 minutes

Cooking time: 15 minutes

Number of servings: 2

Ingredients:

- 1/2 cup quinoa, rinsed

- 1 cup water

- 1 cup almond milk (or any plant-based milk)

- 1 tablespoon maple syrup (or sweetener of choice)

- 1 teaspoon vanilla extract

- Toppings: sliced fruits, nuts, seeds, coconut flakes

Instructions:

1. In a saucepan, combine the quinoa, water, and almond milk.

2. Bring to a boil, then reduce the heat to low, cover, and simmer for 15 minutes or until the quinoa is cooked and fluffy.

3. Remove from heat and stir in the maple syrup and vanilla extract.

4. Divide the cooked quinoa between serving bowls.

5. Top with your choice of sliced fruits, nuts, seeds, and coconut flakes.

6. Drizzle with additional maple syrup if desired.

7. Serve warm and enjoy this wholesome breakfast bowl!

Nutritional info: (Per serving)

- Calories: 300

- Fat: 8g

- Carbohydrates: 50g

- Protein: 10g

Vegan Breakfast Sandwich

Description: A delicious and satisfying sandwich filled with tofu scramble, avocado, and fresh vegetables, perfect for a quick and easy breakfast on the go.

Preparation time: 10 minutes

Cooking time: 10 minutes

Number of servings: 2

Ingredients:

- 1 block firm tofu, drained and pressed

- 1 tablespoon olive oil

- 1/2 teaspoon turmeric

- 1/2 teaspoon cumin

- Salt and pepper to taste

- 4 slices whole grain bread, toasted

- 1 ripe avocado, sliced

- 1 tomato, sliced

- Handful of spinach leaves

- Optional: vegan cheese slices, hot sauce

Instructions:

1. Crumble the pressed tofu into a bowl using your hands or a fork.

2. Heat the olive oil in a skillet over medium heat.

3. Add the crumbled tofu to the skillet and sprinkle with turmeric, cumin, salt, and pepper.

4. Cook for 5-7 minutes, stirring occasionally, until the tofu is heated through and slightly browned.

5. Assemble the sandwiches by layering the tofu scramble, sliced avocado, tomato, and spinach leaves onto the toasted bread slices.

6. Add any optional ingredients such as vegan cheese slices or hot sauce.

7. Top with the remaining bread slices to form sandwiches.

8. Serve immediately, or wrap in foil for a portable breakfast option!

Nutritional info: (Per serving)

- Calories: 350

- Fat: 18g

- Carbohydrates: 30g

- Protein: 15g

Coconut Yogurt with Granola

Description: A creamy and dairy-free yogurt alternative paired with crunchy granola for a satisfying and nutritious breakfast or snack.

Preparation time: 5 minutes

Number of servings: 2

Ingredients:

- 1 cup coconut yogurt (store-bought or homemade)

- 1/2 cup granola (store-bought or homemade)

- Optional toppings: sliced fruits, nuts, seeds, or a drizzle of honey or maple syrup

Instructions:

1. Divide the coconut yogurt evenly between serving bowls.

2. Top with granola and any optional toppings of your choice.

3. Serve immediately and enjoy this delicious and wholesome treat!

Nutritional info: (Per serving)

- Calories: 250

- Fat: 10g

- Carbohydrates: 30g

- Protein: 8g

Banana Walnut Muffins

Description: Moist and flavorful muffins made with ripe bananas and crunchy walnuts, perfect for a quick breakfast or snack.

Preparation time: 15 minutes

Cooking time: 20 minutes

Number of servings: 12 muffins

Ingredients:

- 2 cups all-purpose flour

- 1 teaspoon baking powder

- 1/2 teaspoon baking soda

- 1/4 teaspoon salt

- 1/2 cup coconut oil, melted

- 3/4 cup brown sugar

- 2 ripe bananas, mashed

- 2 flax eggs (2 tablespoons ground flaxseed + 6 tablespoons water)

- 1 teaspoon vanilla extract

- 1/2 cup chopped walnuts

Instructions:

1. Preheat the oven to 350°F (175°C). Line a muffin tin with paper liners or lightly grease with coconut oil.

2. In a large mixing bowl, whisk together the flour, baking powder, baking soda, and salt.

3. In a separate bowl, mix together the melted coconut oil and brown sugar until well combined.

4. Add the mashed bananas, flax eggs, and vanilla extract to the wet ingredients, and mix until smooth.

5. Pour the wet ingredients into the dry ingredients and stir until just combined.

6. Gently fold in the chopped walnuts.

7. Divide the batter evenly among the muffin cups, filling each about 2/3 full.

8. Bake for 18-20 minutes, or until a toothpick inserted into the center of a muffin comes out clean.

9. Remove from the oven and let cool in the pan for 5 minutes before transferring to a wire rack to cool completely.

10. Enjoy these delicious banana walnut muffins warm or at room temperature!

Nutritional info: (Per muffin)

- Calories: 200

- Fat: 10g

- Carbohydrates: 25g

- Protein: 3g

Green Smoothie

Description: A nutrient-packed smoothie featuring leafy greens, fruits, and a touch of sweetness for a refreshing and energizing start to the day.

Preparation time: 5 minutes

Number of servings: 2

Ingredients:

- 2 cups fresh spinach leaves

- 1 ripe banana

- 1/2 cup frozen pineapple chunks

- 1/2 cup frozen mango chunks

- 1 tablespoon chia seeds

- 1 cup coconut water or water

- Optional: honey or maple syrup for extra sweetness

Instructions:

1. Place all the ingredients in a blender.

2. Blend until smooth and creamy, adding more coconut water or water if needed to reach your desired consistency.

3. Taste and add honey or maple syrup if you prefer a sweeter smoothie.

4. Pour into glasses and serve immediately.

5. Enjoy this vibrant and nutritious green smoothie!

Nutritional info: (Per serving)

- Calories: 150

- Fat: 3g

- Carbohydrates: 30g

- Protein: 3g

Sweet Potato Hash

Description: A hearty and flavorful breakfast dish made with sweet potatoes, onions, bell peppers, and spices, perfect for a weekend brunch.

Preparation time: 15 minutes

Cooking time: 20 minutes

Number of servings: 4

Ingredients:

- 2 large sweet potatoes, peeled and diced

- 1 onion, diced

- 1 bell pepper, diced

- 2 cloves garlic, minced

- 2 tablespoons olive oil

- 1 teaspoon smoked paprika

- 1/2 teaspoon cumin

- Salt and pepper to taste

- Fresh parsley or cilantro for garnish

Instructions:

1. Heat the olive oil in a large skillet over medium heat.

2. Add the diced sweet potatoes to the skillet and cook for 5 minutes, stirring occasionally.

3. Add the diced onion, bell pepper, and minced garlic to the skillet. Cook for another 7-8 minutes, or until the sweet potatoes are tender and lightly browned.

4. Stir in the smoked paprika, cumin, salt, and pepper. Mix well to coat the vegetables evenly with the spices.

5. Cook for an additional 2-3 minutes, then remove from heat.

6. Garnish with fresh parsley or cilantro before serving.

7. Enjoy this flavorful sweet potato hash on its own or topped with a fried egg or avocado!

Nutritional info: (Per serving)

- Calories: 200

- Fat: 7g

- Carbohydrates: 30g

- Protein: 3g

Acai Bowl

Description: A refreshing and antioxidant-rich breakfast bowl made with acai puree, topped with granola, fruits, and nuts for a delicious and nutritious treat.

Preparation time: 10 minutes

Number of servings: 2

Ingredients:

- 2 packs frozen acai puree (unsweetened)

- 1 ripe banana

- 1/2 cup frozen mixed berries (strawberries, blueberries, raspberries)

- 1/2 cup almond milk (or any plant-based milk)

- Toppings: granola, sliced fruits, shredded coconut, nuts, seeds

Instructions:

1. In a blender, combine the frozen acai puree, banana, mixed berries, and almond milk.

2. Blend until smooth and creamy, adding more almond milk if needed to achieve a thick and smooth consistency.

3. Divide the acai mixture between serving bowls.

4. Top with granola, sliced fruits, shredded coconut, nuts, and seeds.

5. Serve immediately and enjoy this vibrant and delicious acai bowl!

Nutritional info: (Per serving)

- Calories: 250

- Fat: 10g

- Carbohydrates: 35g

- Protein: 5g

Vegan French Toast

Description: A cruelty-free twist on the classic French toast, made with a rich and creamy batter and cooked until golden brown.

Preparation time: 10 minutes

Cooking time: 10 minutes

Number of servings: 4

Ingredients:

- 8 slices of your favorite bread (preferably slightly stale)

- 1 cup unsweetened almond milk (or any plant-based milk)

- 2 tablespoons flour (all-purpose or whole wheat)

- 1 tablespoon nutritional yeast (optional, for a cheesy flavor)

- 1 tablespoon maple syrup (or sweetener of choice)

- 1 teaspoon vanilla extract

- 1/2 teaspoon ground cinnamon

- Pinch of salt

- Coconut oil or vegan butter for cooking

Instructions:

1. In a shallow dish, whisk together the almond milk, flour, nutritional yeast, maple syrup, vanilla extract, cinnamon, and salt until smooth.

2. Heat a non-stick skillet or griddle over medium heat and lightly grease with coconut oil or vegan butter.

3. Dip each slice of bread into the batter, making sure to coat both sides evenly.

4. Place the coated bread slices onto the preheated skillet or griddle.

5. Cook for 3-4 minutes on each side, or until golden brown and crispy.

6. Serve hot with your favorite toppings such as fresh fruits, maple syrup, or vegan whipped cream.

7. Enjoy this indulgent and delicious vegan French toast!

Nutritional info: (Per serving, without toppings)

- Calories: 200

- Fat: 5g

- Carbohydrates: 35g

- Protein: 5g

Spinach and Mushroom Omelette (using tofu)

Description: A savory and protein-packed omelette made with tofu instead of eggs, filled with nutritious spinach and mushrooms.

Preparation time: 10 minutes

Cooking time: 10 minutes

Number of servings: 2

Ingredients:

- 1 block firm tofu, drained and pressed

- 1 tablespoon olive oil

- 1/2 onion, diced

- 1 cup sliced mushrooms

- 2 cups fresh spinach leaves

- 2 cloves garlic, minced

- 1/2 teaspoon turmeric

- Salt and pepper to taste

- Optional: nutritional yeast for a cheesy flavor

Instructions:

1. Crumble the pressed tofu into a bowl using your hands or a fork.

2. Heat the olive oil in a skillet over medium heat.

3. Add the diced onion to the skillet and sauté until softened, about 3-4 minutes.

4. Add the sliced mushrooms to the skillet and cook until softened and browned, about 5 minutes.

5. Stir in the minced garlic and cook for another 1-2 minutes until fragrant.

6. Add the fresh spinach leaves to the skillet and cook until wilted, about 1-2 minutes.

7. Push the vegetables to one side of the skillet and add the crumbled tofu to the other side.

8. Season the tofu with turmeric, salt, and pepper. Cook for 5-7 minutes, stirring occasionally, until heated through and slightly browned.

9. Optional: sprinkle nutritional yeast over the tofu for a cheesy flavor.

10. Fold the cooked vegetables into the tofu mixture to form the omelette.

11. Cook for another 2-3 minutes, or until the omelette is set and cooked through.

12. Serve hot and enjoy this delicious spinach and mushroom tofu omelette!

Nutritional info: (Per serving)

- Calories: 200

- Fat: 10g

- Carbohydrates: 10g

- Protein: 15g

Vegan Breakfast Tacos

Description: Flavorful and satisfying breakfast tacos filled with scrambled tofu, black beans, avocado, and salsa, perfect for a hearty morning meal.

Preparation time: 15 minutes

Cooking time: 10 minutes

Number of servings: 4

Ingredients:

- 1 block firm tofu, drained and pressed

- 1 tablespoon olive oil

- 1/2 onion, diced

- 1 bell pepper, diced

- 1 teaspoon ground cumin

- 1/2 teaspoon chili powder

- Salt and pepper to taste

- 1 cup cooked black beans

- 8 small corn tortillas, warmed

- 1 ripe avocado, sliced

- Salsa, for serving

- Fresh cilantro, for garnish

Instructions:

1. Crumble the pressed tofu into a bowl using your hands or a fork.

2. Heat the olive oil in a skillet over medium heat.

3. Add the diced onion and bell pepper to the skillet and sauté until softened, about 3-4 minutes.

4. Stir in the crumbled tofu, ground cumin, chili powder, salt, and pepper. Mix well to combine.

5. Cook for 5-7 minutes, stirring occasionally, until the tofu is heated through and slightly browned.

6. Warm the corn tortillas in a dry skillet or microwave.

7. To assemble the tacos, divide the scrambled tofu mixture evenly among the tortillas.

8. Top each taco with black beans, sliced avocado, salsa, and fresh cilantro.

9. Serve immediately and enjoy these delicious vegan breakfast tacos!

Nutritional info: (Per serving, 2 tacos)

- Calories: 300

- Fat: 12g

- Carbohydrates: 35g

- Protein: 12g

Blueberry Almond Butter Toast

Description: A simple yet delicious breakfast or snack option featuring creamy almond butter and fresh blueberries on whole grain toast.

Preparation time: 5 minutes

Number of servings: 2

Ingredients:

- 4 slices whole grain bread, toasted

- 4 tablespoons almond butter

- 1 cup fresh blueberries

- Optional: drizzle of honey or maple syrup

Instructions:

1. Spread 1 tablespoon of almond butter onto each slice of toasted bread.

2. Arrange fresh blueberries on top of the almond butter.

3. Optional: drizzle with honey or maple syrup for added sweetness.

4. Serve immediately and enjoy this quick and nutritious blueberry almond butter toast!

Nutritional info: (Per serving)

- Calories: 250

- Fat: 10g

- Carbohydrates: 35g

- Protein: 8g

Vegan Breakfast Quesadilla

Description: A flavorful and satisfying quesadilla filled with scrambled tofu, black beans, vegetables, and vegan cheese, perfect for a savory breakfast or brunch.

Preparation time: 15 minutes

Cooking time: 10 minutes

Number of servings: 2

Ingredients:

- 1 block firm tofu, drained and pressed

- 1 tablespoon olive oil

- 1/2 onion, diced

- 1 bell pepper, diced

- 1 teaspoon ground cumin

- 1/2 teaspoon chili powder

- Salt and pepper to taste

- 1 cup cooked black beans

- 4 small whole wheat tortillas

- 1/2 cup vegan cheese shreds

- Salsa, for serving

- Fresh cilantro, for garnish

Instructions:

1. Crumble the pressed tofu into a bowl using your hands or a fork.

2. Heat the olive oil in a skillet over medium heat.

3. Add the diced onion and bell pepper to the skillet and sauté until softened, about 3-4 minutes.

4. Stir in the crumbled tofu, ground cumin, chili powder, salt, and pepper. Mix well to combine.

5. Cook for 5-7 minutes, stirring occasionally, until the tofu is heated through and slightly browned.

6. Warm the tortillas in a dry skillet or microwave.

7. To assemble the quesadillas, spread a layer of scrambled tofu mixture onto half of each tortilla.

8. Top with black beans and vegan cheese shreds.

9. Fold the other half of the tortilla over the filling to form a half-moon shape.

10. Heat a skillet over medium heat and lightly grease with olive oil.

11. Cook the quesadillas for 2-3 minutes on each side, or until golden brown and crispy.

12. Serve hot with salsa and fresh cilantro on top.

13. Enjoy these delicious vegan breakfast quesadillas as a satisfying meal any time of day!

Nutritional info: (Per serving, 1 quesadilla)

- Calories: 350

- Fat: 15g

- Carbohydrates: 40g

- Protein: 15g

Vegan Breakfast Hash

Description: A hearty and flavorful breakfast dish made with potatoes, vegetables, and savory seasonings, perfect for a satisfying morning meal.

Preparation time: 15 minutes

Cooking time: 25 minutes

Number of servings: 4

Ingredients:

- 4 medium potatoes, diced

- 1 tablespoon olive oil

- 1/2 onion, diced

- 1 bell pepper, diced

- 1 cup diced mushrooms

- 2 cloves garlic, minced

- 1 teaspoon smoked paprika

- 1/2 teaspoon ground cumin

- Salt and pepper to taste

- Fresh parsley or cilantro for garnish

Instructions:

1. Heat the olive oil in a large skillet over medium heat.

2. Add the diced potatoes to the skillet and cook for 10-15 minutes, stirring occasionally, until tender and golden brown.

3. Add the diced onion, bell pepper, mushrooms, and minced garlic to the skillet. Cook for another 5-7 minutes, or until the vegetables are softened.

4. Stir in the smoked paprika, ground cumin, salt, and pepper. Mix well to coat the vegetables evenly with the spices.

5. Cook for an additional 2-3 minutes, then remove from heat.

6. Garnish with fresh parsley or cilantro before serving.

7. Enjoy this delicious and satisfying vegan breakfast hash on its own or with your favorite toppings!

Nutritional info: (Per serving)

- Calories: 200

- Fat: 5g

- Carbohydrates: 35g

- Protein: 5g

Oatmeal with Berries and Nuts

Description: A comforting and nutritious breakfast bowl made with hearty oats, sweet berries, and crunchy nuts, perfect for a cozy morning meal.

Preparation time: 5 minutes

Cooking time: 5 minutes

Number of servings: 2

Ingredients:

- 1 cup rolled oats

- 2 cups water or plant-based milk

- 1 cup mixed berries (strawberries, blueberries, raspberries)

- 1/4 cup chopped nuts (almonds, walnuts, pecans)

- Maple syrup or honey for drizzling (optional)

Instructions:

1. In a saucepan, bring the water or plant-based milk to a boil.

2. Stir in the rolled oats and reduce heat to low. Cook for 5 minutes, stirring occasionally, until the oats are creamy and tender.

3. Divide the cooked oats between serving bowls.

4. Top with mixed berries and chopped nuts.

5. Optional: drizzle with maple syrup or honey for added sweetness.

6. Serve hot and enjoy this delicious oatmeal with berries and nuts!

Nutritional info: (Per serving)

- Calories: 250

- Fat: 10g

- Carbohydrates: 35g

- Protein: 7g

Vegan Breakfast Biscuits and Gravy

Description: A comforting and satisfying breakfast dish featuring fluffy biscuits smothered in a creamy vegan gravy, perfect for a weekend brunch.

Preparation time: 20 minutes

Cooking time: 20 minutes

Number of servings: 4

Ingredients:

For the Biscuits:

- 2 cups all-purpose flour

- 1 tablespoon baking powder

- 1/2 teaspoon baking soda

- 1/2 teaspoon salt

- 1/2 cup vegan butter, cold and cubed

- 3/4 cup almond milk (or any plant-based milk)

For the Gravy:

- 2 tablespoons olive oil

- 1/4 cup all-purpose flour

- 2 cups almond milk (or any plant-based milk)

- 1 teaspoon garlic powder

- 1 teaspoon onion powder

- Salt and pepper to taste

Instructions:

1. Preheat the oven to 425°F (220°C). Line a baking sheet with parchment paper.

2. In a large mixing bowl, whisk together the flour, baking powder, baking soda, and salt.

3. Add the cold vegan butter to the flour mixture and use a pastry cutter or fork to cut it into the flour until the mixture resembles coarse crumbs.

4. Pour in the almond milk and stir until just combined, being careful not to overmix.

5. Turn the dough out onto a lightly floured surface and gently knead it a few times until it comes together.

6. Roll out the dough to about 1/2 inch thickness and use a biscuit cutter to cut out biscuits. Place the biscuits onto the prepared baking sheet.

7. Bake for 12-15 minutes, or until the biscuits are golden brown and cooked through.

8. While the biscuits are baking, prepare the gravy. Heat the olive oil in a skillet over medium heat.

9. Whisk in the flour and cook for 1-2 minutes, stirring constantly, until lightly golden brown.

10. Slowly pour in the almond milk, whisking constantly to prevent lumps from forming.

11. Stir in the garlic powder, onion powder, salt, and pepper. Cook for another 5-7 minutes, or until the gravy has thickened to your desired consistency.

12. Serve the warm biscuits topped with the creamy vegan gravy.

13. Enjoy these delicious vegan breakfast biscuits and gravy as a comforting morning meal!

Nutritional info: (Per serving, 1 biscuit with gravy)

- Calories: 350

- Fat: 15g

- Carbohydrates: 45g

- Protein: 8g

Vegan Breakfast Cookies

Description: A wholesome and portable breakfast option packed with oats, nuts, seeds, and dried fruits, perfect for busy mornings on the go.

Preparation time: 15 minutes

Cooking time: 15 minutes

Number of servings: 12 cookies

Ingredients:

- 2 ripe bananas, mashed

- 1/4 cup coconut oil, melted

- 1/4 cup maple syrup or agave nectar

- 1 teaspoon vanilla extract

- 2 cups rolled oats

- 1/2 cup chopped nuts (almonds, walnuts, pecans)

- 1/4 cup seeds (pumpkin seeds, sunflower seeds)

- 1/4 cup dried fruits (raisins, cranberries, chopped apricots)

- Pinch of salt

Instructions:

1. Preheat the oven to 350°F (175°C). Line a baking sheet with parchment paper.

2. In a large mixing bowl, combine the mashed bananas, melted coconut oil, maple syrup, and vanilla extract.

3. Stir in the rolled oats, chopped nuts, seeds, dried fruits, and a pinch of salt. Mix until well combined.

4. Scoop out about 2 tablespoons of the dough and shape it into a cookie on the prepared baking sheet. Repeat with the remaining dough, spacing the cookies a few inches apart.

5. Flatten each cookie slightly with the back of a spoon or your fingers.

6. Bake for 12-15 minutes, or until the cookies are golden brown and set.

7. Remove from the oven and let cool on the baking sheet for 5 minutes before transferring to a wire rack to cool completely.

8. Enjoy these nutritious vegan breakfast cookies as a quick and satisfying morning treat!

Nutritional info: (Per serving, 1 cookie)

- Calories: 150

- Fat: 8g

- Carbohydrates: 18g

- Protein: 3g

Peanut Butter Banana Toast

Description: A simple yet delicious breakfast option featuring creamy peanut butter and sliced bananas on whole grain toast, perfect for a quick and satisfying morning meal.

Preparation time: 5 minutes

Number of servings: 2

Ingredients:

- 4 slices whole grain bread, toasted

- 4 tablespoons peanut butter

- 2 ripe bananas, sliced

- Optional: drizzle of honey or maple syrup

Instructions:

1. Spread 1 tablespoon of peanut butter onto each slice of toasted bread.

2. Arrange sliced bananas on top of the peanut butter.

3. Optional: drizzle with honey or maple syrup for added sweetness.

4. Serve immediately and enjoy this quick and nutritious peanut butter banana toast!

Nutritional info: (Per serving)

- Calories: 250

- Fat: 10g

- Carbohydrates: 35g

- Protein: 8g

Chapter 4

Midday Meals for Sustained Energy

Quinoa Salad

Description: A refreshing and nutritious salad featuring quinoa, colorful vegetables, and a zesty dressing.

Preparation time: 15 minutes

Cooking time: 15 minutes

Number of servings: 4

Ingredients:

- 1 cup quinoa

- 2 cups water or vegetable broth

- 1 cucumber, diced

- 1 bell pepper, diced

- 1 cup cherry tomatoes, halved

- 1/4 cup red onion, finely chopped

- 1/4 cup fresh parsley, chopped

- 1/4 cup olive oil

- 2 tablespoons lemon juice

- 2 cloves garlic, minced

- Salt and pepper to taste

Instructions:

1. Rinse the quinoa under cold water. In a pot, bring the water or vegetable broth to a boil. Add quinoa, cover, and reduce heat to low.

Simmer for about 15 minutes or until the quinoa is cooked and the water is absorbed.

2. Fluff the quinoa with a fork and let it cool.

3. In a large bowl, combine the cooked quinoa, cucumber, bell pepper, cherry tomatoes, red onion, and parsley.

4. In a small bowl, whisk together olive oil, lemon juice, garlic, salt, and pepper to make the dressing.

5. Pour the dressing over the quinoa salad and toss until well combined.

6. Serve chilled or at room temperature.

    Nutritional info: (Serving size: 1/4 of the recipe)

- Calories: 280

- Fat: 14g

- Carbohydrates: 32g

- Protein: 7g

Lentil Soup

Description: Hearty and comforting lentil soup packed with vegetables and savory spices.

Preparation time: 10 minutes

Cooking time: 30 minutes

Number of servings: 6

Ingredients:

- 1 cup dry lentils, rinsed

- 6 cups vegetable broth

- 1 onion, diced

- 2 carrots, diced

- 2 celery stalks, diced

- 2 cloves garlic, minced

- 1 teaspoon cumin

- 1 teaspoon paprika

- 1/2 teaspoon turmeric

- Salt and pepper to taste

- 2 tablespoons olive oil

- Fresh parsley for garnish (optional)

Instructions:

1. In a large pot, heat olive oil over medium heat. Add onion, carrots, and celery. Sauté until vegetables are softened, about 5 minutes.

2. Add garlic, cumin, paprika, and turmeric. Cook for another 2 minutes until fragrant.

3. Add lentils and vegetable broth to the pot. Bring to a boil, then reduce heat to low and simmer for 20-25 minutes, or until lentils are tender.

4. Season with salt and pepper to taste.

5. Serve hot, garnished with fresh parsley if desired.

Nutritional info: (Serving size: 1/6 of the recipe)

- Calories: 180

- Fat: 4g

- Carbohydrates: 28g

- Protein: 10g

Chickpea Salad Sandwich

Description: A delicious and satisfying sandwich filled with a creamy chickpea salad.

Preparation time: 15 minutes

Cooking time: 0 minutes

Number of servings: 4

Ingredients:

- 1 can (15 ounces) chickpeas, drained and rinsed

- 1/4 cup vegan mayonnaise

- 1 tablespoon Dijon mustard

- 2 tablespoons lemon juice

- 1/4 cup celery, finely chopped

- 2 tablespoons red onion, finely chopped

- Salt and pepper to taste

- 8 slices whole grain bread

- Lettuce leaves

- Tomato slices

- Avocado slices (optional)

Instructions:

1. In a mixing bowl, mash the chickpeas with a fork until coarse.

2. Add vegan mayonnaise, Dijon mustard, lemon juice, celery, and red onion to the mashed chickpeas. Stir until well combined.

3. Season with salt and pepper to taste.

4. To assemble the sandwiches, spread the chickpea salad onto one slice of bread. Top with lettuce, tomato, and avocado slices if desired. Cover with another slice of bread.

5. Repeat with the remaining ingredients to make the remaining sandwiches.

6. Serve immediately or wrap tightly for later.

    Nutritional info: (Serving size: 1 sandwich)

- Calories: 320

- Fat: 10g

- Carbohydrates: 47g

- Protein: 12g

Vegan Sushi Rolls

Description: Colorful and flavorful sushi rolls filled with fresh vegetables and creamy avocado.

Preparation time: 30 minutes

Cooking time: 0 minutes

Number of servings: 4 rolls

Ingredients:

- 1 cup sushi rice

- 2 cups water

- 4 nori seaweed sheets

- 1 avocado, sliced

- 1/2 cucumber, julienned

- 1 carrot, julienned

- 1/2 red bell pepper, julienned

- Soy sauce, for serving

- Pickled ginger, for serving

- Wasabi, for serving

Instructions:

1. Rinse sushi rice under cold water until the
    water runs clear. Cook rice according to
    package instructions.

2. Place a nori sheet on a bamboo sushi mat.
    Spread a thin layer of cooked rice over the nori,
    leaving a 1-inch border at the top.

3. Arrange avocado slices, cucumber, carrot, and
    bell pepper in the center of the rice.

4. Using the bamboo mat, roll the sushi tightly
    from bottom to top, applying gentle pressure
    as you roll.

5. Moisten the top border of the nori with a little
    water to seal the roll.

6. Repeat with the remaining nori sheets and
    ingredients.

7. Using a sharp knife, slice each roll into 6-8
    pieces.

8. Serve sushi rolls with soy sauce, pickled ginger,
    and wasabi.

Nutritional info: (Serving size: 1 roll)

- Calories: 180

- Fat: 5g

- Carbohydrates: 30g

- Protein: 4g

Buddha Bowl

Description: A nourishing bowl filled with a
variety of plant-based ingredients, perfect for a
satisfying meal.

Preparation time: 20 minutes

Cooking time: 20 minutes

Number of servings: 4

Ingredients:

- 1 cup quinoa

- 2 cups water or vegetable broth

- 1 sweet potato, diced

- 1 cup broccoli florets

- 1 cup chickpeas, cooked

- 1 avocado, sliced

- 1/4 cup hummus

- 2 tablespoons tahini

- 2 tablespoons lemon juice

- Salt and pepper to taste

- Fresh cilantro for garnish (optional)

Instructions:

1. Rinse quinoa under cold water. In a pot, bring water or vegetable broth to a boil. Add quinoa, cover, and reduce heat to low. Simmer for about 15 minutes or until quinoa is cooked and water is absorbed.

2. Preheat oven to 400°F (200°C). On a baking sheet, arrange sweet potato and broccoli in a single layer. Drizzle with olive oil, salt, and pepper. Roast for 20 minutes or until tender and golden brown.

3. In a small bowl, whisk together tahini, lemon juice, salt, and pepper to make the dressing.

4. To assemble the Buddha bowls, divide cooked quinoa among serving bowls. Top with roasted

sweet potato, broccoli, chickpeas, avocado slices, and hummus.

5. Drizzle tahini dressing over the bowls.

6. Garnish with fresh cilantro if desired.

7. Serve immediately.

Nutritional info: (Serving size: 1 bowl)

- Calories: 450

- Fat: 20g

- Carbohydrates: 55g

- Protein: 15g

Black Bean Tacos

Description: Flavorful and satisfying tacos filled with seasoned black beans and fresh toppings.

Preparation time: 15 minutes

Cooking time: 15 minutes

Number of servings: 4 (2 tacos per serving)

Ingredients:

- 1 can (15 ounces) black beans, drained and rinsed

- 1 tablespoon olive oil

- 1 onion, diced

- 2 cloves garlic, minced

- 1 teaspoon chili powder

- 1/2 teaspoon cumin

- Salt and pepper to taste

- 8 small corn or flour tortillas

- Toppings: shredded lettuce, diced tomatoes, diced avocado, salsa, cilantro, lime wedges

Instructions:

1. In a skillet, heat olive oil over medium heat. Add onion and garlic, sauté until softened, about 3 minutes.

2. Add black beans, chili powder, cumin, salt, and pepper. Cook for another 5 minutes, stirring occasionally.

3. Warm tortillas according to package instructions.

4. To assemble tacos, spoon black bean mixture onto each tortilla. Top with lettuce, tomatoes, avocado, salsa, and cilantro.

5. Serve with lime wedges for squeezing over the tacos.

Nutritional info: (Serving size: 2 tacos)

- Calories: 320

- Fat: 8g

- Carbohydrates: 52g

- Protein: 12g

Hummus Wrap

Description: A quick and easy wrap featuring creamy hummus and fresh vegetables.

Preparation time: 10 minutes

Cooking time: 0 minutes

Number of servings: 2

Ingredients:

- 2 large whole wheat wraps or tortillas

- 1/2 cup hummus

- 1 cup mixed salad greens

- 1/2 cucumber, sliced

- 1/2 bell pepper, sliced

- 1/4 cup shredded carrots

- 1/4 cup alfalfa sprouts

- Salt and pepper to taste

Instructions:

1. Lay out the wraps on a clean surface.

2. Spread hummus evenly over each wrap.

3. Layer salad greens, cucumber slices, bell pepper slices, shredded carrots, and alfalfa sprouts on top of the hummus.

4. Season with salt and pepper to taste.

5. Roll up the wraps tightly, folding in the sides as you go.

6. Cut each wrap in half diagonally.

7. Serve immediately or wrap tightly for later.

   Nutritional info: (Serving size: 1 wrap)

- Calories: 300

- Fat: 12g

- Carbohydrates: 38g

- Protein: 10g

Mediterranean Couscous Salad

Description: A vibrant salad featuring couscous, cherry tomatoes, cucumbers, olives, and feta cheese, tossed in a lemon herb dressing.

Preparation time: 15 minutes

Cooking time: 10 minutes

Number of servings: 4

Ingredients:

- 1 cup couscous

- 1 1/4 cups vegetable broth or water

- 1 cup cherry tomatoes, halved

- 1/2 cucumber, diced

- 1/4 cup Kalamata olives, pitted and sliced

- 2 tablespoons red onion, finely chopped

- 1/4 cup crumbled feta cheese

- 2 tablespoons fresh parsley, chopped

- 2 tablespoons fresh mint, chopped

- 2 tablespoons olive oil

- 2 tablespoons lemon juice

- Salt and pepper to taste

Instructions:

1. In a saucepan, bring vegetable broth or water to a boil. Stir in couscous, cover, and remove from heat. Let stand for 5 minutes, then fluff with a fork and let cool.

2. In a large bowl, combine cooked couscous, cherry tomatoes, cucumber, olives, red onion, feta cheese, parsley, and mint.

3. In a small bowl, whisk together olive oil, lemon juice, salt, and pepper to make the dressing.

4. Pour the dressing over the salad and toss until well combined.

5. Serve immediately or refrigerate until ready to serve.

Nutritional info: (Serving size: 1/4 of the recipe)

- Calories: 280

- Fat: 10g

- Carbohydrates: 40g

- Protein: 8g

Veggie Stir-Fry with Tofu

Description: A colorful and nutritious stir-fry featuring tofu and an assortment of fresh vegetables in a savory sauce.

Preparation time: 15 minutes

Cooking time: 15 minutes

Number of servings: 4

Ingredients:

- 1 block (14 ounces) firm tofu, drained and cubed

- 2 tablespoons soy sauce

- 1 tablespoon sesame oil

- 1 tablespoon cornstarch

- 1 tablespoon vegetable oil

- 2 cloves garlic, minced

- 1 tablespoon ginger, minced

- 1 bell pepper, sliced

- 1 cup broccoli florets

- 1 carrot, julienned

- 1/2 cup snow peas

- 1/4 cup vegetable broth

- 2 tablespoons hoisin sauce

- Cooked rice or noodles, for serving

Instructions:

1. In a bowl, combine tofu, soy sauce, sesame oil, and cornstarch. Toss to coat tofu evenly.

2. Heat vegetable oil in a large skillet or wok over medium-high heat. Add tofu and cook until golden brown on all sides, about 5-7 minutes. Remove tofu from skillet and set aside.

3. In the same skillet, add garlic and ginger. Sauté for 1 minute until fragrant.

4. Add bell pepper, broccoli, carrot, and snow peas to the skillet. Cook for 5-7 minutes until vegetables are tender-crisp.

5. In a small bowl, whisk together vegetable broth and hoisin sauce. Pour over the vegetables in the skillet.

6. Return tofu to the skillet and toss everything together until well coated in the sauce.

7. Serve hot over cooked rice or noodles.

Nutritional info: (Serving size: 1/4 of the recipe, without rice or noodles)

- Calories: 220

- Fat: 12g

- Carbohydrates: 14g

- Protein: 16g

Sweet Potato and Black Bean Enchiladas

Description: Flavorful enchiladas filled with roasted sweet potatoes, black beans, and spices, topped with enchilada sauce and melted cheese.

Preparation time: 20 minutes

Cooking time: 30 minutes

Number of servings: 6

Ingredients:

- 2 large sweet potatoes, peeled and diced

- 1 can (15 ounces) black beans, drained and rinsed

- 1 tablespoon olive oil

- 1 onion, diced

- 2 cloves garlic, minced

- 1 teaspoon chili powder

- 1/2 teaspoon cumin

- Salt and pepper to taste

- 12 small corn tortillas

- 2 cups enchilada sauce

- 1 cup shredded Mexican blend cheese

- Fresh cilantro for garnish (optional)

- Sour cream or Greek yogurt for serving (optional)

Instructions:

1. Preheat oven to 400°F (200°C). Place diced sweet potatoes on a baking sheet, drizzle with olive oil, and sprinkle with chili powder, cumin, salt, and pepper. Toss to coat evenly. Roast for 20 minutes or until tender.

2. In a skillet, heat olive oil over medium heat. Add onion and garlic, sauté until softened, about 3 minutes.

3. Add black beans to the skillet, along with the roasted sweet potatoes. Stir to combine and cook for another 5 minutes. Remove from heat.

4. Warm corn tortillas in the microwave or on a skillet until soft and pliable.

5. Spread a thin layer of enchilada sauce on the bottom of a 9x13-inch baking dish.

6. Spoon sweet potato and black bean mixture onto each tortilla, roll up tightly, and place seam-side down in the baking dish.

7. Pour remaining enchilada sauce over the rolled tortillas, making sure they are all evenly coated.

8. Sprinkle shredded cheese over the top of the enchiladas.

9. Bake in the preheated oven for 15 minutes or until the cheese is melted and bubbly.

10. Garnish with fresh cilantro if desired and serve hot with sour cream or Greek yogurt.

Nutritional info: (Serving size: 2 enchiladas)

- Calories: 420

- Fat: 12g

- Carbohydrates: 65g

- Protein: 16g

Vegan Caesar Salad

Description: A refreshing and flavorful Caesar salad made with crisp romaine lettuce, crunchy croutons, and a creamy vegan Caesar dressing.

Preparation time: 15 minutes

Cooking time: 10 minutes

Number of servings: 4

Ingredients:

For the dressing:

- 1/2 cup raw cashews, soaked in water for at least 2 hours

- 2 tablespoons lemon juice

- 2 tablespoons nutritional yeast

- 1 tablespoon Dijon mustard

- 2 cloves garlic, minced

- 1/4 cup water

- Salt and pepper to taste

For the salad:

- 1 large head romaine lettuce, chopped

- 1 cup cherry tomatoes, halved

- 1/4 cup sliced red onion

- 1/2 cup croutons (check for vegan options)

Instructions:

1. To make the dressing, drain the soaked cashews and add them to a blender along with lemon juice, nutritional yeast, Dijon mustard, garlic, water, salt, and pepper. Blend until smooth and creamy. Add more water if needed to reach your desired consistency.

2. In a large bowl, combine chopped romaine lettuce, cherry tomatoes, and sliced red onion.

3. Pour the dressing over the salad and toss until well coated.

4. Top with croutons just before serving.

5. Serve immediately.

Nutritional info: (Serving size: 1/4 of the salad with dressing)

- Calories: 180

- Fat: 10g

- Carbohydrates: 20g

- Protein: 7g

Portobello Mushroom Burger

Description: A hearty and satisfying burger featuring grilled portobello mushrooms marinated in savory flavors, topped with your favorite burger fixings.

Preparation time: 10 minutes

Cooking time: 10 minutes

Number of servings: 4

Ingredients:

- 4 large portobello mushroom caps, stems removed

- 1/4 cup balsamic vinegar

- 2 tablespoons soy sauce

- 2 cloves garlic, minced

- 2 tablespoons olive oil

- Salt and pepper to taste

- 4 burger buns

- Burger toppings of your choice (lettuce, tomato, onion, avocado, etc.)

Instructions:

1. In a shallow dish, whisk together balsamic vinegar, soy sauce, minced garlic, olive oil, salt, and pepper to make the marinade.

2. Place portobello mushroom caps in the marinade, turning to coat evenly. Let marinate for at least 30 minutes.

3. Preheat grill or grill pan over medium-high heat. Remove mushrooms from marinade and grill for 4-5 minutes per side, or until tender and slightly charred.

4. Toast burger buns on the grill for 1-2 minutes, if desired.

5. Assemble burgers by placing grilled portobello mushrooms on the bottom half of each bun.

Top with your favorite burger toppings and the other half of the bun.

6. Serve immediately.

Nutritional info: (Serving size: 1 burger)

- Calories: 200

- Fat: 8g

- Carbohydrates: 28g

- Protein: 7g

Vegan Pasta Primavera

Description: A colorful and flavorful pasta dish loaded with fresh vegetables and tossed in a light and tangy vegan sauce.

Preparation time: 15 minutes

Cooking time: 15 minutes

Number of servings: 4

Ingredients:

- 8 ounces pasta of your choice

- 2 tablespoons olive oil

- 2 cloves garlic, minced

- 1 small yellow onion, thinly sliced

- 1 bell pepper, thinly sliced

- 1 zucchini, thinly sliced

- 1 cup cherry tomatoes, halved

- 1 cup broccoli florets

- 1/4 cup vegetable broth

- 2 tablespoons lemon juice

- 1/4 cup nutritional yeast (optional)

- Salt and pepper to taste

- Fresh basil for garnish (optional)

Instructions:

1. Cook pasta according to package instructions until al dente. Drain and set aside.

2. In a large skillet, heat olive oil over medium heat. Add minced garlic and sliced onion, sauté until softened, about 3 minutes.

3. Add bell pepper, zucchini, cherry tomatoes, and broccoli florets to the skillet. Cook for 5-7 minutes until vegetables are tender-crisp.

4. Stir in vegetable broth, lemon juice, nutritional yeast (if using), salt, and pepper. Cook for another 2 minutes.

5. Add cooked pasta to the skillet and toss until well coated with the sauce.

6. Serve hot, garnished with fresh basil if desired.

   Nutritional info: (Serving size: 1/4 of the
   pasta)

- Calories: 300

- Fat: 8g

- Carbohydrates: 50g

- Protein: 10g

Falafel Wrap

Description: A flavorful and satisfying wrap filled with crispy falafel, fresh vegetables, and creamy tahini sauce.

Preparation time: 20 minutes

Cooking time: 10 minutes

Number of servings: 4

Ingredients:

For the falafel:

- 1 can (15 ounces) chickpeas, drained and rinsed

- 1/4 cup fresh parsley, chopped

- 2 cloves garlic, minced

- 1 teaspoon ground cumin

- 1 teaspoon ground coriander

- 1/2 teaspoon salt

- 1/4 teaspoon black pepper

- 1 tablespoon lemon juice

- 2 tablespoons all-purpose flour or chickpea flour

- 2 tablespoons olive oil, for frying

For the wrap:

- 4 large whole wheat wraps or tortillas

- 1 cup shredded lettuce

- 1 cucumber, sliced

- 1 tomato, sliced

- 1/4 cup sliced red onion

- 1/4 cup hummus

- 1/4 cup tahini sauce (store-bought or homemade)

- Fresh parsley for garnish (optional)

Instructions:

1. In a food processor, combine chickpeas, parsley, garlic, cumin, coriander, salt, pepper, and lemon juice. Pulse until mixture is finely chopped and holds together when pressed.

2. Transfer the falafel mixture to a bowl and stir
    in flour until well combined.

3. Shape falafel mixture into small patties.

4. Heat olive oil in a skillet over medium heat. Fry
    falafel patties for 3-4 minutes per side until
    golden brown and crispy. Drain on paper
    towels.

5. Warm wraps or tortillas according to package
    instructions.

6. Spread hummus evenly over each wrap. Layer
    shredded lettuce, cucumber slices, tomato
    slices, red onion slices, and falafel patties on
    top.

7. Drizzle tahini sauce over the filling.

8. Roll up the wraps tightly, folding in the sides as
    you go.

9. Cut each wrap in half diagonally.

10. Garnish with fresh parsley if desired.

11. Serve immediately or wrap tightly for later.

Nutritional info: (Serving size: 1 wrap)

- Calories: 350

- Fat: 15g

- Carbohydrates: 45g

- Protein: 12g

Stuffed Bell Peppers with Rice and Beans

Description: Bell peppers stuffed with a flavorful mixture of rice, beans, vegetables, and spices, baked to perfection.

Preparation time: 20 minutes

Cooking time: 40 minutes

Number of servings: 4

Ingredients:

- 4 large bell peppers, tops removed and seeds removed

- 1 cup cooked rice

- 1 can (15 ounces) black beans, drained and rinsed

- 1 cup corn kernels

- 1/2 cup diced tomatoes

- 1/4 cup diced red onion

- 2 cloves garlic, minced

- 1 teaspoon chili powder

- 1/2 teaspoon cumin

- Salt and pepper to taste

- 1 cup shredded vegan cheese (optional)

- Fresh cilantro for garnish (optional)

Instructions:

1. Preheat oven to 375°F (190°C). Place bell peppers in a baking dish.

2. In a large bowl, combine cooked rice, black beans, corn kernels, diced tomatoes, red onion, minced garlic, chili powder, cumin, salt, and pepper.

3. Spoon the rice and bean mixture into each bell pepper until they are filled to the top.

4. If using vegan cheese, sprinkle it over the stuffed bell peppers.

5. Cover the baking dish with foil and bake in the preheated oven for 30 minutes.

6. Remove foil and bake for an additional 10 minutes, or until the peppers are tender and the filling is heated through.

7. Garnish with fresh cilantro if desired.

8. Serve hot.

Nutritional info: (Serving size: 1 stuffed bell pepper)

- Calories: 280

- Fat: 2g

- Carbohydrates: 55g

- Protein: 12g

Vegan Pad Thai

Description: A delicious and vegan version of the classic Thai noodle dish, packed with vegetables and tofu, and tossed in a tangy and savory sauce.

Preparation time: 20 minutes

Cooking time: 15 minutes

Number of servings: 4

Ingredients:

- 8 ounces rice noodles

- 2 tablespoons tamarind paste

- 2 tablespoons soy sauce

- 1 tablespoon maple syrup or agave nectar

- 1 tablespoon rice vinegar

- 1 tablespoon lime juice

- 2 tablespoons peanut oil or vegetable oil

- 2 cloves garlic, minced

- 1 block (14 ounces) extra-firm tofu, drained and pressed, cut into cubes

- 1 cup shredded carrots

- 1 cup bean sprouts

- 4 green onions, sliced

- 1/4 cup chopped peanuts (optional)

- Fresh cilantro for garnish (optional)

- Lime wedges for serving

Instructions:

1. Cook rice noodles according to package instructions until al dente. Drain and set aside.

2. In a small bowl, whisk together tamarind paste, soy sauce, maple syrup, rice vinegar, and lime juice to make the sauce. Set aside.

3. Heat peanut oil in a large skillet or wok over medium-high heat. Add minced garlic and cubed tofu. Cook until tofu is golden brown on all sides, about 5-7 minutes.

4. Add shredded carrots, bean sprouts, and sliced green onions to the skillet. Cook for another 3-4 minutes until vegetables are tender-crisp.

5. Add cooked rice noodles and sauce to the skillet. Toss everything together until well coated in the sauce and heated through.

6. Serve hot, garnished with chopped peanuts, fresh cilantro, and lime wedges.

Nutritional info: (Serving size: 1/4 of the recipe)

- Calories: 380

- Fat: 15g

- Carbohydrates: 50g

- Protein: 15g

Veggie Spring Rolls with Peanut Dipping Sauce

Description: Fresh and crispy spring rolls filled with colorful vegetables and served with a creamy peanut dipping sauce.

Preparation time: 30 minutes

Cooking time: 0 minutes

Number of servings: 4 (2 rolls per serving)

Ingredients:

For the spring rolls:

- 8 rice paper wrappers

- 2 cups shredded lettuce

- 1 cucumber, julienned

- 1 carrot, julienned

- 1 bell pepper, julienned

- 1/2 cup fresh cilantro leaves

- 1/2 cup fresh mint leaves

- 1/2 cup cooked rice vermicelli noodles (optional)

For the peanut dipping sauce:

- 1/4 cup creamy peanut butter

- 2 tablespoons soy sauce

- 1 tablespoon maple syrup or agave nectar

- 1 tablespoon lime juice

- 1 clove garlic, minced

- 2-4 tablespoons water, as needed

Instructions:

1. Prepare all the vegetables and herbs for the spring rolls and arrange them on a plate.

2. Fill a shallow dish with warm water. Dip one rice paper wrapper into the water for a few seconds until it softens.

3. Place the softened rice paper wrapper on a clean, flat surface.

4. Layer a small amount of shredded lettuce, julienned cucumber, carrot, bell pepper,

cilantro leaves, mint leaves, and rice vermicelli noodles (if using) on the bottom third of the rice paper wrapper.

5. Fold the bottom of the wrapper over the filling, then fold in the sides, and roll tightly to enclose the filling.

6. Repeat with the remaining rice paper wrappers and filling ingredients.

7. To make the peanut dipping sauce, whisk together peanut butter, soy sauce, maple syrup, lime juice, minced garlic, and water until smooth and creamy. Add more water as needed to reach your desired consistency.

8. Serve spring rolls immediately with peanut dipping sauce on the side.

Nutritional info: (Serving size: 2 spring rolls with dipping sauce)

- Calories: 250

- Fat: 10g

- Carbohydrates: 35g

- Protein: 8g

Coconut Curry with Vegetables

Description: A fragrant and creamy coconut curry loaded with assorted vegetables and aromatic spices, served over rice.

Preparation time: 15 minutes

Cooking time: 25 minutes

Number of servings: 4

Ingredients:

- 1 tablespoon coconut oil or vegetable oil

- 1 onion, diced

- 2 cloves garlic, minced

- 1 tablespoon grated ginger

- 2 tablespoons curry powder

- 1 teaspoon ground turmeric

- 1 can (14 ounces) coconut milk

- 1 cup vegetable broth

- 2 cups assorted vegetables (such as bell pepper, broccoli, carrots, and peas)

- Salt and pepper to taste

- Cooked rice for serving

- Fresh cilantro for garnish (optional)

Instructions:

1. Heat coconut oil in a large skillet or pot over medium heat. Add diced onion and cook until softened, about 5 minutes.

2. Add minced garlic, grated ginger, curry powder, and ground turmeric to the skillet. Cook for another 2 minutes until fragrant.

3. Stir in coconut milk and vegetable broth, and bring to a simmer.

4. Add assorted vegetables to the skillet and simmer for 15-20 minutes, or until vegetables are tender.

5. Season with salt and pepper to taste.

6. Serve hot over cooked rice, garnished with fresh cilantro if desired.

Nutritional info: (Serving size: 1/4 of the curry with rice)

- Calories: 350

- Fat: 20g

- Carbohydrates: 35g

- Protein: 8g

Vegan Chili

Description: A hearty and flavorful chili made with beans, vegetables, and savory spices, perfect for a comforting and satisfying meal.

Preparation time: 15 minutes

Cooking time: 30 minutes

Number of servings: 6

Ingredients:

- 1 tablespoon olive oil

- 1 onion, diced

- 2 cloves garlic, minced

- 1 bell pepper, diced

- 1 zucchini, diced

- 1 carrot, diced

- 1 can (15 ounces) black beans, drained and rinsed

- 1 can (15 ounces) kidney beans, drained and rinsed

- 1 can (15 ounces) diced tomatoes

- 2 cups vegetable broth

- 2 tablespoons tomato paste

- 1 tablespoon chili powder

- 1 teaspoon ground cumin

- 1 teaspoon smoked paprika

- Salt and pepper to taste

- Optional toppings: diced avocado, chopped cilantro, vegan sour cream, sliced green onions

Instructions:

1. Heat olive oil in a large pot over medium heat. Add diced onion and minced garlic, sauté until softened, about 5 minutes.

2. Add diced bell pepper, zucchini, and carrot to the pot. Cook for another 5 minutes until vegetables are tender.

3. Stir in black beans, kidney beans, diced tomatoes, vegetable broth, tomato paste, chili powder, ground cumin, smoked paprika, salt, and pepper.

4. Bring chili to a simmer and cook for 20-25 minutes, stirring occasionally, until flavors are well combined and vegetables are tender.

5. Taste and adjust seasoning if needed.

6. Serve hot, garnished with diced avocado, chopped cilantro, vegan sour cream, and sliced green onions if desired.

Nutritional info: (Serving size: 1/6 of the chili)

- Calories: 250

- Fat: 5g

- Carbohydrates: 45g

- Protein: 12g

Mediterranean Quinoa Stuffed Tomatoes

Description: Juicy tomatoes stuffed with a flavorful mixture of quinoa, chickpeas, olives, and herbs, baked until tender.

Preparation time: 20 minutes

Cooking time: 25 minutes

Number of servings: 4

Ingredients:

- 4 large tomatoes

- 1 cup cooked quinoa

- 1 can (15 ounces) chickpeas, drained and rinsed

- 1/4 cup Kalamata olives, pitted and chopped

- 1/4 cup sun-dried tomatoes, chopped

- 2 tablespoons fresh parsley, chopped

- 2 tablespoons fresh basil, chopped

- 2 tablespoons olive oil

- 1 tablespoon lemon juice

- Salt and pepper to taste

- 1/4 cup breadcrumbs (optional)

- Vegan feta cheese, crumbled (optional)

Instructions:

1. Preheat oven to 375°F (190°C). Slice off the tops of the tomatoes and scoop out the seeds and pulp to create a hollow cavity.

2. In a large bowl, combine cooked quinoa, chickpeas, chopped olives, chopped sun-dried tomatoes, chopped parsley, chopped basil, olive oil, lemon juice, salt, and pepper.

3. Stuff each tomato with the quinoa mixture, pressing gently to pack it in.

4. If using breadcrumbs, sprinkle them over the top of each stuffed tomato for a crunchy topping.

5. Place stuffed tomatoes in a baking dish and bake in the preheated oven for 20-25 minutes, or until tomatoes are tender and slightly wrinkled.

6. If desired, sprinkle vegan feta cheese over the top of each stuffed tomato before serving.

7. Serve hot.

Nutritional info: (Serving size: 1 stuffed tomato)

- Calories: 220

- Fat: 8g

- Carbohydrates: 30g

- Protein: 9g

Vegan Pizza with Loads of Veggies

Description: A delicious homemade pizza topped with an assortment of colorful vegetables and vegan cheese, perfect for a satisfying meal.

Preparation time: 30 minutes

Cooking time: 15 minutes

Number of servings: 4

Ingredients:

- 1 pre-made pizza dough (store-bought or homemade)

- 1/2 cup marinara sauce

- 1 cup vegan mozzarella cheese, shredded

- Assorted vegetables (such as bell peppers, mushrooms, onions, tomatoes, spinach, olives, etc.), sliced or diced

- Fresh basil leaves for garnish

- Red pepper flakes for sprinkling (optional)

Instructions:

1. Preheat oven to 425°F (220°C). If using a pizza stone, place it in the oven to preheat.

2. Roll out the pizza dough on a lightly floured surface to your desired thickness.

3. Transfer the rolled-out dough to a pizza pan or preheated pizza stone.

4. Spread marinara sauce evenly over the dough, leaving a small border around the edges.

5. Sprinkle vegan mozzarella cheese over the sauce.

6. Arrange assorted vegetables over the cheese.

7. Bake pizza in the preheated oven for 12-15 minutes, or until the crust is golden brown and the cheese is melted and bubbly.

8. Remove pizza from the oven and let it cool slightly.

9. Garnish with fresh basil leaves and sprinkle with red pepper flakes if desired.

10. Slice and serve hot.

Nutritional info: (Serving size: 1/4 of the pizza)

- Calories: 300

- Fat: 10g

- Carbohydrates: 45g

- Protein: 10g

Tofu Banh Mi Sandwich

Description: A vegan twist on the classic Vietnamese banh mi sandwich, featuring marinated tofu, crunchy vegetables, and tangy pickled carrots and daikon, all served on a crusty baguette.

Preparation time: 30 minutes

Cooking time: 10 minutes

Number of servings: 4

Ingredients:

For the marinated tofu:

- 1 block (14 ounces) firm tofu, pressed and sliced

- 1/4 cup soy sauce

- 2 tablespoons rice vinegar

- 2 tablespoons maple syrup or agave nectar

- 2 cloves garlic, minced

- 1 teaspoon grated ginger

- 1 teaspoon sesame oil

- Salt and pepper to taste

For the sandwich:

- 4 small baguettes or sandwich rolls

- Vegan mayonnaise

- Sliced cucumber

- Sliced jalapeños

- Pickled carrots and daikon (store-bought or homemade)

- Fresh cilantro sprigs

Instructions:

1. In a shallow dish, whisk together soy sauce, rice vinegar, maple syrup, minced garlic, grated ginger, sesame oil, salt, and pepper to make the marinade.

2. Place sliced tofu in the marinade, turning to coat evenly. Let marinate for at least 20 minutes.

3. Preheat grill or grill pan over medium-high heat. Grill marinated tofu slices for 3-4 minutes per side, or until golden brown and heated through.

4. Slice baguettes or sandwich rolls in half lengthwise.

5. Spread vegan mayonnaise on the bottom half of each baguette.

6. Layer grilled tofu slices, sliced cucumber, sliced jalapeños, pickled carrots and daikon, and fresh cilantro sprigs on top of the mayonnaise.

7. Close the sandwiches with the top half of the baguettes.

8. Serve immediately.

Nutritional info: (Serving size: 1 sandwich)

- Calories: 350

- Fat: 10g

- Carbohydrates: 45g

- Protein: 15g

Kale and Avocado Salad with Lemon Tahini Dressing

Description: A nutritious and flavorful salad featuring hearty kale, creamy avocado, and a zesty lemon tahini dressing.

Preparation time: 15 minutes

Cooking time: 0 minutes

Number of servings: 4

Ingredients:

For the salad:

- 1 bunch kale, stems removed and leaves torn into bite-sized pieces

- 1 avocado, diced

- 1/4 cup sliced almonds, toasted

- 1/4 cup dried cranberries or raisins

- 2 tablespoons hemp seeds (optional)

- Salt and pepper to taste

For the lemon tahini dressing:

- 1/4 cup tahini

- 2 tablespoons lemon juice

- 2 tablespoons water

- 1 tablespoon maple syrup or agave nectar

- 1 clove garlic, minced

- Salt and pepper to taste

Instructions:

1. In a large bowl, massage kale leaves with a bit of olive oil for a few minutes to soften them.

2. Add diced avocado, toasted sliced almonds, dried cranberries or raisins, and hemp seeds (if using) to the bowl with kale.

3. In a small bowl, whisk together tahini, lemon juice, water, maple syrup, minced garlic, salt, and pepper to make the dressing. Add more water if needed to reach your desired consistency.

4. Drizzle the dressing over the salad and toss until well coated.

5. Season with additional salt and pepper to taste, if needed.

6. Serve immediately.

    Nutritional info: (Serving size: 1/4 of the salad with dressing)

- Calories: 250

- Fat: 18g

- Carbohydrates: 20g

- Protein: 8g

Vegan BLT Sandwich

Description: A plant-based version of the classic BLT sandwich, featuring smoky tempeh bacon, crisp lettuce, ripe tomatoes, and creamy avocado.

Preparation time: 20 minutes

Cooking time: 10 minutes

Number of servings: 4

Ingredients:

For the tempeh bacon:

- 1 package (8 ounces) tempeh, thinly sliced

- 3 tablespoons soy sauce

- 1 tablespoon maple syrup or agave nectar

- 1 teaspoon liquid smoke

- 1/2 teaspoon smoked paprika

- 1/4 teaspoon garlic powder

- 1/4 teaspoon black pepper

- 1 tablespoon vegetable oil

For the sandwich:

- 8 slices whole grain bread, toasted

- Vegan mayonnaise

- Lettuce leaves

- Sliced tomatoes

- Sliced avocado

Instructions:

1. In a shallow dish, whisk together soy sauce, maple syrup, liquid smoke, smoked paprika, garlic powder, and black pepper to make the marinade for the tempeh bacon.

2. Add thinly sliced tempeh to the marinade, turning to coat evenly. Let marinate for at least 10 minutes.

3. Heat vegetable oil in a skillet over medium heat. Add marinated tempeh slices to the skillet and cook for 3-4 minutes per side, or until golden brown and crispy.

4. Assemble sandwiches by spreading vegan mayonnaise on one side of each slice of toasted bread.

5. Layer lettuce leaves, sliced tomatoes, avocado slices, and cooked tempeh bacon on top of the mayonnaise.

6. Close the sandwiches with the remaining slices of toasted bread.

7. Slice sandwiches in half diagonally and serve immediately.

   Nutritional info: (Serving size: 1 sandwich)

- Calories: 350

- Fat: 15g

- Carbohydrates: 40g

- Protein: 15g

Vegan Macaroni and Cheese

Description: Creamy and cheesy macaroni and cheese made with a rich and velvety cashew-based sauce, perfect for a comforting meal.

Preparation time: 20 minutes

Cooking time: 20 minutes

Number of servings: 6

Ingredients:

- 12 ounces elbow macaroni or pasta of your choice

- 1 cup raw cashews, soaked in water for at least 2 hours

- 1 cup unsweetened almond milk or other plant-based milk

- 1/4 cup nutritional yeast

- 2 tablespoons lemon juice

- 1 tablespoon white miso paste

- 1 teaspoon garlic powder

- 1 teaspoon onion powder

- 1/2 teaspoon turmeric powder (for color)

- Salt and pepper to taste

- Chopped fresh parsley for garnish (optional)

Instructions:

1. Cook macaroni or pasta according to package instructions until al dente. Drain and set aside.

2. In a blender, combine soaked cashews, almond milk, nutritional yeast, lemon juice, white miso paste, garlic powder, onion powder, turmeric

powder, salt, and pepper. Blend until smooth and creamy.

3. In a large pot, heat the cashew sauce over medium heat until heated through.

4. Add cooked macaroni or pasta to the pot with the sauce. Stir until well coated and heated through.

5. Taste and adjust seasoning if needed.

6. Serve hot, garnished with chopped fresh parsley if desired.

Nutritional info: (Serving size: 1/6 of the macaroni and cheese)

- Calories: 350

- Fat: 10g

- Carbohydrates: 50g

- Protein: 12g

Chapter 5

Healthy Plant-Based Snacks

Edamame with Sea Salt

Description: A simple and nutritious snack featuring steamed edamame beans sprinkled with sea salt.

Preparation time: 5 minutes

Cooking time: 5 minutes

Number of servings: 4

Ingredients:

- 2 cups frozen edamame in pods

- Sea salt, to taste

Instructions:

1. Bring a pot of water to a boil.

2. Add the frozen edamame pods and cook for about 5 minutes, until tender.

3. Drain the edamame and transfer to a serving bowl.

4. Sprinkle with sea salt to taste.

5. Toss to coat evenly and serve warm.

Nutritional info:

- Calories per serving: 100

- Protein: 8g

- Carbohydrates: 9g

- Fat: 4g

Sliced Apples with Almond Butter

Description: Crisp apple slices paired with creamy almond butter for a satisfying and healthy snack.

Preparation time: 5 minutes

Number of servings: 2

Ingredients:

- 2 medium apples, cored and sliced
- 4 tablespoons almond butter

Instructions:

1. Arrange the apple slices on a plate.
2. Place almond butter in a small bowl for dipping.

3. Serve alongside the apple slices for a delicious snack.

Nutritional info:

- Calories per serving: 210

- Protein: 5g

- Carbohydrates: 27g

- Fat: 11g

Guacamole and Veggie Sticks

Description: Freshly made guacamole paired with colorful vegetable sticks for a flavorful and nutritious snack.

Preparation time: 10 minutes

Number of servings: 6

Ingredients:

- 3 ripe avocados, peeled and mashed

- 1 tomato, diced

- 1/4 cup red onion, finely chopped

- 1/4 cup cilantro, chopped

- 1 lime, juiced

- Salt and pepper, to taste

- Assorted vegetable sticks (carrots, celery, bell peppers, etc.)

Instructions:

1. In a mixing bowl, combine mashed avocados, diced tomato, red onion, cilantro, lime juice, salt, and pepper. Mix well.

2. Adjust seasoning to taste.

3. Serve the guacamole with assorted vegetable sticks for dipping.

Nutritional info:

- Calories per serving: 160

- Protein: 3g

- Carbohydrates: 11g

- Fat: 13g

Roasted Chickpeas

Description: Crispy roasted chickpeas seasoned with savory spices for a flavorful snack.

Preparation time: 5 minutes

Cooking time: 30 minutes

Number of servings: 4

Ingredients:

- 2 cans (15 oz each) chickpeas, drained and rinsed

- 2 tablespoons olive oil

- 1 teaspoon ground cumin

- 1 teaspoon smoked paprika

- 1/2 teaspoon garlic powder

- Salt, to taste

Instructions:

1. Preheat the oven to 400°F (200°C).

2. Pat the chickpeas dry with a paper towel and remove any loose skins.

3. In a bowl, toss chickpeas with olive oil, cumin, paprika, garlic powder, and salt until evenly coated.

4. Spread the seasoned chickpeas in a single layer on a baking sheet.

5. Roast in the preheated oven for 25-30 minutes, stirring halfway through, until crispy and golden brown.

6. Remove from the oven and let cool slightly before serving.

Nutritional info:

- Calories per serving: 230

- Protein: 10g

- Carbohydrates: 29g

- Fat: 9g

Trail Mix with Nuts, Seeds, and Dried Fruit

Description: A customizable blend of nuts, seeds, and dried fruit for a convenient and energy-boosting snack.

Preparation time: 5 minutes

Number of servings: 8

Ingredients:

- 1 cup almonds

- 1 cup cashews

- 1 cup pumpkin seeds

- 1 cup dried cranberries

- 1/2 cup raisins

- 1/2 cup dried apricots, chopped

Instructions:

1. In a large bowl, combine almonds, cashews, pumpkin seeds, dried cranberries, raisins, and chopped dried apricots.

2. Mix well to evenly distribute ingredients.

3. Transfer the trail mix to an airtight container for storage.

4. Enjoy as a convenient on-the-go snack!

Nutritional info:

- Calories per serving: 250

- Protein: 8g

- Carbohydrates: 25g

- Fat: 15g

Popcorn (Air-Popped) with Nutritional Yeast

Description: Light and crunchy air-popped popcorn seasoned with savory nutritional yeast for a flavorful twist.

Preparation time: 5 minutes

Cooking time: 5 minutes

Number of servings: 4

Ingredients:

- 1/2 cup popcorn kernels
- 2 tablespoons nutritional yeast
- Salt, to taste

Instructions:

1. Air-pop the popcorn kernels according to your popcorn maker's instructions.

2. Transfer the popped popcorn to a large bowl.

3. Sprinkle nutritional yeast and salt over the popcorn while still warm.

4. Toss gently to coat evenly.

5. Serve immediately for a delicious and nutritious snack.

Nutritional info:

- Calories per serving: 80

- Protein: 3g

- Carbohydrates: 15g

- Fat: 1g

Rice Cakes with Avocado and Tomato Slices

Description: Crispy rice cakes topped with creamy avocado and juicy tomato slices for a light and refreshing snack.

Preparation time: 5 minutes

Number of servings: 2

Ingredients:

- 2 rice cakes

- 1 ripe avocado, sliced

- 1 tomato, sliced

- Salt and pepper, to taste

Instructions:

1. Place rice cakes on a serving plate.

2. Top each rice cake with slices of avocado and tomato.

3. Season with salt and pepper to taste.

4. Serve immediately for a quick and satisfying snack.

Nutritional info:

- Calories per serving: 150

- Protein: 3g

- Carbohydrates: 19g

- Fat: 7g

Carrot Sticks with Hummus

Description: Crunchy carrot sticks served with creamy hummus for a satisfying and nutritious snack.

Preparation time: 5 minutes

Number of servings: 4

Ingredients:

- 4 large carrots, peeled and cut into sticks

- 1 cup hummus

Instructions:

1. Arrange carrot sticks on a serving platter.

2. Place hummus in a bowl for dipping.

3. Serve carrot sticks with hummus for a delicious and healthy snack.

Nutritional info:

- Calories per serving: 120

- Protein: 5g

- Carbohydrates: 15g

- Fat: 5g

Frozen Grapes

Description: Sweet and refreshing frozen grapes make for a delightful and healthy frozen treat.

Preparation time: 5 minutes

Number of servings: 4

Ingredients:

- 2 cups grapes, washed and stemmed

Instructions:

1. Spread the washed and stemmed grapes in a single layer on a baking sheet.

2. Place the baking sheet in the freezer and freeze for at least 2 hours, or until the grapes are completely frozen.

3. Transfer the frozen grapes to an airtight container for storage.

4. Serve the frozen grapes straight from the freezer for a refreshing snack.

Nutritional info:

- Calories per serving: 60

- Protein: 1g

- Carbohydrates: 15g

- Fat: 0g

Vegan Energy Balls

Description: Nutrient-packed energy balls made with wholesome ingredients for a convenient and energizing snack.

Preparation time: 15 minutes

Number of servings: 12

Ingredients:

- 1 cup rolled oats

- 1/2 cup almond butter

- 1/4 cup maple syrup

- 1/4 cup shredded coconut

- 1/4 cup chopped nuts (such as almonds, walnuts, or cashews)

- 1/4 cup dried fruit (such as raisins, dates, or apricots)

- 1 tablespoon chia seeds (optional)

- 1 teaspoon vanilla extract

- Pinch of salt

Instructions:

1. In a large mixing bowl, combine rolled oats, almond butter, maple syrup, shredded coconut, chopped nuts, dried fruit, chia seeds (if using), vanilla extract, and a pinch of salt.

2. Mix until well combined and the mixture holds together when pressed.

3. Roll the mixture into small balls, about 1 inch in diameter, and place them on a baking sheet lined with parchment paper.

4. Refrigerate the energy balls for at least 30 minutes to firm up.

5. Once chilled, transfer the energy balls to an airtight container for storage.

6. Enjoy as a convenient and nutritious snack anytime!

Nutritional info:

- Calories per serving (1 energy ball): 120

- Protein: 3g

- Carbohydrates: 12g

- Fat: 7g

Veggie Chips (Baked)

Description: Crispy and flavorful baked veggie chips made from a variety of colorful vegetables.

Preparation time: 15 minutes

Cooking time: 20 minutes

Number of servings: 4

Ingredients:

- 2 large carrots, peeled

- 2 medium beets, peeled

- 1 large sweet potato, peeled

- 2 tablespoons olive oil

- Salt and pepper, to taste

Instructions:

1. Preheat the oven to 375°F (190°C) and line a baking sheet with parchment paper.

2. Using a mandoline slicer or sharp knife, thinly slice the carrots, beets, and sweet potato into rounds.

3. In a large bowl, toss the sliced vegetables with olive oil, salt, and pepper until evenly coated.

4. Arrange the vegetable slices in a single layer on the prepared baking sheet.

5. Bake in the preheated oven for 20-25 minutes, flipping halfway through, until the chips are crisp and lightly golden.

6. Remove from the oven and let cool slightly before serving.

Nutritional info:

- Calories per serving: 120

- Protein: 2g

- Carbohydrates: 15g

- Fat: 7g

Almonds and Dark Chocolate

Description: A delicious and satisfying snack featuring crunchy almonds paired with rich dark chocolate.

Preparation time: 2 minutes

Number of servings: 4

Ingredients:

- 1 cup almonds

- 4 ounces dark chocolate, chopped

Instructions:

1. Divide the almonds and dark chocolate evenly into 4 small bowls or snack containers.

2. Enjoy a handful of almonds along with a piece of dark chocolate for a delightful snack.

Nutritional info:

- Calories per serving: 200

- Protein: 5g

- Carbohydrates: 10g

- Fat: 15g

Celery Sticks with Peanut Butter and Raisins (Ants on a Log)

Description: Classic childhood snack featuring crisp celery sticks filled with creamy peanut butter and topped with sweet raisins.

Preparation time: 5 minutes

Number of servings: 4

Ingredients:

- 4 celery stalks, washed and trimmed

- 1/4 cup peanut butter

- 1/4 cup raisins

Instructions:

1. Spread peanut butter evenly onto each celery stalk.

2. Press raisins into the peanut butter along the length of the celery stalks.

3. Serve immediately for a fun and nutritious snack reminiscent of "ants on a log."

Nutritional info:

- Calories per serving: 150

- Protein: 4g

- Carbohydrates: 10g

- Fat: 11g

Kale Chips

Description: Crispy and flavorful kale chips seasoned with savory spices for a healthy and satisfying snack.

Preparation time: 10 minutes

Cooking time: 15 minutes

Number of servings: 4

Ingredients:

- 1 bunch kale, stems removed and torn into bite-sized pieces

- 2 tablespoons olive oil

- 1 teaspoon garlic powder

- 1 teaspoon paprika

- Salt, to taste

Instructions:

1. Preheat the oven to 325°F (160°C) and line a baking sheet with parchment paper.

2. In a large bowl, toss the kale pieces with olive oil, garlic powder, paprika, and salt until evenly coated.

3. Spread the seasoned kale in a single layer on the prepared baking sheet.

4. Bake in the preheated oven for 12-15 minutes, or until the kale is crispy but not burnt.

5. Remove from the oven and let cool slightly before serving.

Nutritional info:

- Calories per serving: 80

- Protein: 3g

- Carbohydrates: 5g

- Fat: 6g

Vegan Yogurt with Berries

Description: Creamy vegan yogurt topped with fresh berries for a refreshing and nutritious snack.

Preparation time: 2 minutes

Number of servings: 2

Ingredients:

- 1 cup vegan yogurt (such as almond or coconut yogurt)

- 1 cup mixed berries (such as strawberries, blueberries, and raspberries)

Instructions:

1. Divide the vegan yogurt into serving bowls.

2. Top each bowl of yogurt with an equal amount of mixed berries.

3. Serve immediately for a delicious and satisfying snack.

Nutritional info:

- Calories per serving: 120

- Protein: 3g

- Carbohydrates: 15g

- Fat: 5g

Cucumber Slices with Tahini

Description: Refreshing cucumber slices paired with creamy tahini for a light and flavorful snack.

Preparation time: 5 minutes

Number of servings: 4

Ingredients:

- 1 large cucumber, washed and sliced

- 1/4 cup tahini

Instructions:

1. Arrange cucumber slices on a serving platter.

2. Drizzle tahini over the cucumber slices.

3. Serve immediately for a refreshing and satisfying snack.

Nutritional info:

- Calories per serving: 60

- Protein: 2g

- Carbohydrates: 4g

- Fat: 5g

Homemade Granola Bars

Description: Wholesome and customizable granola bars packed with oats, nuts, seeds, and dried fruit for a nutritious snack on the go.

Preparation time: 15 minutes

Cooking time: 20 minutes

Number of servings: 12

Ingredients:

- 2 cups rolled oats

- 1/2 cup nuts (such as almonds, walnuts, or pecans), chopped

- 1/4 cup seeds (such as pumpkin or sunflower seeds)

- 1/4 cup dried fruit (such as raisins, cranberries, or apricots), chopped

- 1/4 cup honey or maple syrup

- 1/4 cup nut butter (such as almond or peanut butter)

- 1 tablespoon coconut oil, melted

- 1 teaspoon vanilla extract

- Pinch of salt

Instructions:

1. Preheat the oven to 350°F (175°C) and line a baking dish with parchment paper.

2. In a large bowl, combine rolled oats, chopped nuts, seeds, and dried fruit.

3. In a separate microwave-safe bowl, combine honey or maple syrup, nut butter, melted coconut oil, vanilla extract, and a pinch of salt.

Microwave for 30 seconds, or until the mixture is smooth and well combined.

4. Pour the wet mixture over the dry ingredients and stir until evenly coated.

5. Transfer the mixture to the prepared baking dish and press down firmly to flatten.

6. Bake in the preheated oven for 20-25 minutes, or until golden brown and set.

7. Remove from the oven and let cool completely before cutting into bars.

8. Once cooled, slice into bars and store in an airtight container for up to one week.

Nutritional info:

- Calories per serving: 180

- Protein: 5g

- Carbohydrates: 20g

- Fat: 10g

Roasted Seaweed Snacks

Description: Crispy and savory roasted seaweed sheets seasoned with salt for a light and flavorful snack.

Preparation time: 5 minutes

Cooking time: 10 minutes

Number of servings: 4

Ingredients:

- 4 sheets roasted seaweed

- Salt, to taste

Instructions:

1. Preheat the oven to 325°F (160°C) and line a baking sheet with parchment paper.

2. Place the seaweed sheets on the prepared baking sheet.

3. Sprinkle salt lightly over the seaweed sheets.

4. Bake in the preheated oven for 8-10 minutes, or until the seaweed is crisp.

5. Remove from the oven and let cool before serving.

Nutritional info:

- Calories per serving: 10

- Protein: 1g

- Carbohydrates: 1g

- Fat: 0g

Rice Crackers with Avocado and Sliced Radishes

Description: Crunchy rice crackers topped with creamy avocado and crisp sliced radishes for a satisfying and nutritious snack.

Preparation time: 5 minutes

Number of servings: 2

Ingredients:

- 6 rice crackers

- 1 ripe avocado, mashed

- 4 radishes, thinly sliced

Instructions:

1. Spread mashed avocado evenly onto each rice cracker.

2. Top each rice cracker with sliced radishes.

3. Serve immediately for a tasty and wholesome
    snack.

Nutritional info:

- Calories per serving: 150

- Protein: 3g

- Carbohydrates: 15g

- Fat: 9g

Frozen Banana Slices Dipped in Dark Chocolate

Description: Creamy banana slices dipped in rich dark chocolate for a delicious and satisfying frozen treat.

Preparation time: 15 minutes

Freezing time: 2 hours

Number of servings: 4

Ingredients:

- 2 bananas, peeled and sliced

- 4 ounces dark chocolate, chopped

- Optional toppings: chopped nuts, shredded coconut, sprinkles

Instructions:

1. Line a baking sheet with parchment paper.

2. Arrange banana slices on the prepared baking sheet and place in the freezer for 1 hour.

3. In a microwave-safe bowl, melt the dark chocolate in 30-second intervals, stirring until smooth.

4. Dip each frozen banana slice into the melted chocolate, coating evenly.

5. Place the chocolate-covered banana slices back on the parchment paper-lined baking sheet.

6. Optional: Sprinkle with chopped nuts, shredded coconut, or sprinkles before the chocolate sets.

7. Return the baking sheet to the freezer and freeze for an additional hour, or until the chocolate is firm.

8. Once frozen, transfer the banana slices to an airtight container for storage.

9. Serve the frozen banana slices straight from the freezer for a delightful snack.

Nutritional info:

- Calories per serving: 120

- Protein: 2g

- Carbohydrates: 15g

- Fat: 7g

Vegan Cheese and Crackers

Description: Vegan cheese paired with crispy crackers for a savory and satisfying snack.

Preparation time: 5 minutes

Number of servings: 4

Ingredients:

- 1 cup vegan cheese, sliced or cubed

- 16 crackers of your choice

Instructions:

1. Arrange vegan cheese slices or cubes on a serving platter.

2. Place crackers alongside the vegan cheese.

3. Serve immediately for a delicious vegan snack.

Nutritional info:

- Calories per serving: 150

- Protein: 4g

- Carbohydrates: 10g

- Fat: 9g

Mixed Berries

Description: A colorful assortment of fresh mixed berries for a refreshing and nutritious snack.

Preparation time: 2 minutes

Number of servings: 4

Ingredients:

- 2 cups mixed berries (such as strawberries, blueberries, raspberries, and blackberries)

Instructions:

1. Rinse the mixed berries under cold water and pat dry with a paper towel.
2. Arrange the mixed berries on a serving platter or divide them into individual bowls.

3. Serve immediately for a flavorful and healthy snack.

Nutritional info:

- Calories per serving: 60

- Protein: 1g

- Carbohydrates: 15g

- Fat: 0g

Beet Chips

Description: Crispy and vibrant beet chips seasoned with salt for a flavorful and colorful snack.

Preparation time: 10 minutes

Cooking time: 25 minutes

Number of servings: 4

Ingredients:

- 2 large beets, peeled and thinly sliced

- 2 tablespoons olive oil

- Salt, to taste

Instructions:

1. Preheat the oven to 325°F (160°C) and line a baking sheet with parchment paper.

2. In a large bowl, toss the beet slices with olive oil until evenly coated.

3. Arrange the beet slices in a single layer on the prepared baking sheet.

4. Sprinkle salt lightly over the beet slices.

5. Bake in the preheated oven for 20-25 minutes, or until the beet chips are crisp.

6. Remove from the oven and let cool before serving.

Nutritional info:

- Calories per serving: 60

- Protein: 1g

- Carbohydrates: 5g

- Fat: 4g

Stuffed Mini Bell Peppers with Hummus

Description: Mini bell peppers stuffed with creamy hummus for a colorful and flavorful snack.

Preparation time: 10 minutes

Number of servings: 4

Ingredients:

- 12 mini bell peppers, halved and seeded

- 1 cup hummus

Instructions:

1. Fill each mini bell pepper half with a dollop of hummus.

2. Arrange the stuffed mini bell peppers on a serving platter.

3. Serve immediately for a tasty and nutritious snack.

Nutritional info:

- Calories per serving: 100

- Protein: 4g

- Carbohydrates: 10g

- Fat: 6g

Pistachios

Description: Crunchy and flavorful pistachios for a satisfying and nutritious snack.

Preparation time: 2 minutes

Number of servings: 4

Ingredients:

- 1 cup pistachios, shelled

Instructions:

1. Divide the pistachios into individual servings.
2. Enjoy as a convenient and healthy snack.

Nutritional info:

- Calories per serving: 160

- Protein: 6g

- Carbohydrates: 8g

- Fat: 13g

Chapter 6

Creative Dinner Ideas

Veggie Stir-Fry with Tofu

Description: A colorful and flavorful dish packed with vegetables and tofu, stir-fried to perfection.

Preparation time: 15 minutes

Cooking time: 15 minutes

Number of servings: 4

Ingredients:

- 1 block of firm tofu, drained and cubed

- Assorted vegetables (such as bell peppers, broccoli, carrots, and snap peas), sliced

- 3 cloves garlic, minced

- 2 tablespoons soy sauce

- 1 tablespoon sesame oil

- 1 tablespoon vegetable oil

- 1 teaspoon ginger, minced

- Cooked rice or noodles, for serving

Instructions:

1. Heat vegetable oil in a large skillet over medium-high heat. Add tofu cubes and cook until golden brown on all sides. Remove tofu from skillet and set aside.

2. In the same skillet, add sesame oil and sauté garlic and ginger until fragrant.

3. Add sliced vegetables to the skillet and stir-fry until tender-crisp.

4. Return tofu to the skillet, pour soy sauce over the tofu and vegetables, and stir to combine.

5. Serve over cooked rice or noodles.

Nutritional info: (per serving)

- Calories: 250

- Protein: 15g

- Carbohydrates: 20g

- Fat: 12g

Vegan Shepherd's Pie

Description: A comforting and hearty dish made with savory lentils and topped with creamy mashed potatoes.

Preparation time: 20 minutes

Cooking time: 40 minutes

Number of servings: 6

Ingredients:

- 1 cup dried lentils

- 2 cups vegetable broth

- 1 onion, diced

- 2 carrots, diced

- 2 cloves garlic, minced

- 1 cup frozen peas

- 2 tablespoons tomato paste

- 1 teaspoon dried thyme

- Salt and pepper, to taste

- 4 large potatoes, peeled and diced

- 1/4 cup non-dairy milk

- 2 tablespoons vegan butter

- 1 tablespoon nutritional yeast (optional)

Instructions:

1. Preheat oven to 375°F (190°C).

2. In a large pot, combine lentils and vegetable broth. Bring to a boil, then reduce heat and simmer for 20 minutes, or until lentils are tender.

3. In a separate skillet, sauté onion, carrots, and garlic until softened.

4. Add cooked lentils, frozen peas, tomato paste, dried thyme, salt, and pepper to the skillet. Cook for an additional 5 minutes.

5. Meanwhile, boil the diced potatoes until fork-tender. Drain and mash with non-dairy milk, vegan butter, nutritional yeast (if using), salt, and pepper.

6. Transfer the lentil mixture to a baking dish and spread mashed potatoes evenly over the top.

7. Bake for 20-25 minutes, or until the mashed potatoes are lightly golden.

Nutritional info: (per serving)

- Calories: 320

- Protein: 12g

- Carbohydrates: 55g

- Fat: 6g

Quinoa Stuffed Bell Peppers

Description: Bell peppers filled with a flavorful mixture of quinoa, vegetables, and spices.

Preparation time: 15 minutes

Cooking time: 35 minutes

Number of servings: 4

Ingredients:

- 4 large bell peppers, halved and seeds removed

- 1 cup quinoa, cooked

- 1 onion, diced

- 2 cloves garlic, minced

- 1 cup diced tomatoes

- 1 cup black beans, drained and rinsed

- 1 cup corn kernels

- 1 teaspoon cumin

- 1 teaspoon chili powder

- Salt and pepper, to taste

- 1/2 cup shredded vegan cheese (optional)

Instructions:

1. Preheat oven to 375°F (190°C).

2. In a skillet, sauté onion and garlic until softened.

3. Add diced tomatoes, black beans, corn, cumin, chili powder, salt, and pepper to the skillet. Cook for 5 minutes.

4. Stir in cooked quinoa and cook for an additional 2 minutes.

5. Stuff each bell pepper half with the quinoa mixture and place in a baking dish.

6. If desired, sprinkle shredded vegan cheese over the stuffed peppers.

7. Cover the baking dish with foil and bake for 25 minutes. Remove foil and bake for an additional 10 minutes, or until peppers are tender.

Nutritional info: (per serving)

- Calories: 280

- Protein: 11g

- Carbohydrates: 50g

- Fat: 4g

Vegan Pad Thai

Description: A classic Thai dish made with rice noodles, tofu, and a tangy tamarind sauce.

Preparation time: 20 minutes

Cooking time: 15 minutes

Number of servings: 4

Ingredients:

- 8 oz rice noodles

- 1 block of firm tofu, drained and cubed

- 2 tablespoons vegetable oil

- 2 cloves garlic, minced

- 1 cup broccoli florets

- 1 bell pepper, thinly sliced

- 2 carrots, julienned

- 1 cup bean sprouts

- 3 green onions, chopped

- 1/4 cup chopped peanuts (optional)

For the sauce:

- 3 tablespoons soy sauce

- 2 tablespoons tamarind paste

- 2 tablespoons maple syrup

- 1 tablespoon rice vinegar

- 1 teaspoon sriracha (optional)

Instructions:

1. Cook rice noodles according to package instructions. Drain and set aside.

2. In a small bowl, whisk together soy sauce, tamarind paste, maple syrup, rice vinegar, and sriracha to make the sauce.

3. Heat vegetable oil in a large skillet over medium-high heat. Add tofu cubes and cook

until golden brown on all sides. Remove tofu from skillet and set aside.

4. In the same skillet, sauté garlic, broccoli, bell pepper, and carrots until tender-crisp.

5. Add cooked rice noodles, tofu, bean sprouts, green onions, and the prepared sauce to the skillet. Toss everything together until heated through.

6. Serve hot, garnished with chopped peanuts if desired.

Nutritional info: (per serving)

- Calories: 380

- Protein: 12g

- Carbohydrates: 55g

- Fat: 14g

Black Bean and Quinoa Salad

Description: A refreshing and protein-packed salad featuring black beans, quinoa, and a zesty lime dressing.

Preparation time: 15 minutes

Cooking time: 20 minutes (for quinoa, if not pre-cooked)

Number of servings: 4

Ingredients:

- 1 cup quinoa, cooked

- 1 can (15 oz) black beans, drained and rinsed

- 1 cup cherry tomatoes, halved

- 1/2 red onion, diced

- 1 bell pepper, diced

- 1/4 cup chopped cilantro

- 2 tablespoons lime juice

- 2 tablespoons olive oil

- 1 teaspoon cumin

- Salt and pepper, to taste

Instructions:

1. In a large bowl, combine cooked quinoa, black beans, cherry tomatoes, red onion, bell pepper, and cilantro.

2. In a small bowl, whisk together lime juice, olive oil, cumin, salt, and pepper to make the dressing.

3. Pour the dressing over the salad and toss to combine.

4. Chill in the refrigerator for at least 30 minutes before serving to allow the flavors to meld.

Nutritional info: (per serving)

- Calories: 320

- Protein: 14g

- Carbohydrates: 45g

- Fat: 10g

Lentil and Vegetable Soup

Description: A hearty and nutritious soup made with lentils, vegetables, and aromatic spices.

Preparation time: 15 minutes

Cooking time: 40 minutes

Number of servings: 6

Ingredients:

- 1 cup dried green lentils

- 1 onion, diced

- 2 carrots, diced

- 2 celery stalks, diced

- 3 cloves garlic, minced

- 1 can (15 oz) diced tomatoes

- 6 cups vegetable broth

- 1 teaspoon cumin

- 1 teaspoon smoked paprika

- Salt and pepper, to taste

- Fresh parsley, for garnish (optional)

Instructions:

1. In a large pot, sauté onion, carrots, celery, and garlic until softened.

2. Add dried lentils, diced tomatoes, vegetable broth, cumin, smoked paprika, salt, and pepper to the pot. Bring to a boil.

3. Reduce heat and simmer for 30 minutes, or until lentils are tender.

4. Taste and adjust seasonings if needed.

5. Serve hot, garnished with fresh parsley if desired.

Nutritional info: (per serving)

- Calories: 220

- Protein: 12g

- Carbohydrates: 35g

- Fat: 2g

Vegan Fajitas

Description: Flavorful and colorful fajitas made with marinated vegetables and served with tortillas.

Preparation time: 20 minutes

Cooking time: 15 minutes

Number of servings: 4

Ingredients:

- 2 bell peppers, sliced

- 1 onion, sliced

- 1 zucchini, sliced

- 1 yellow squash, sliced

- 1 tablespoon olive oil

- 2 tablespoons fajita seasoning

- 8 small tortillas

- Guacamole, salsa, and vegan sour cream, for serving (optional)

Instructions:

1. In a large bowl, toss sliced bell peppers, onion, zucchini, and yellow squash with olive oil and fajita seasoning until well coated.

2. Heat a large skillet or grill pan over medium-high heat. Add the marinated vegetables and cook for 8-10 minutes, or until vegetables are tender and slightly charred.

3. Warm tortillas according to package instructions.

4. Serve grilled vegetables with warm tortillas and desired toppings such as guacamole, salsa, and vegan sour cream.

Nutritional info: (per serving, excluding toppings)

- Calories: 250

- Protein: 5g

- Carbohydrates: 35g

- Fat: 10g

Zucchini Noodles with Marinara Sauce

Description: A light and healthy alternative to traditional pasta, made with zucchini noodles and topped with marinara sauce.

Preparation time: 10 minutes

Cooking time: 10 minutes

Number of servings: 2

Ingredients:

- 2 large zucchinis, spiralized into noodles

- 2 cups marinara sauce (store-bought or homemade)

- 2 tablespoons olive oil

- 2 cloves garlic, minced

- Salt and pepper, to taste

- Vegan Parmesan cheese, for serving (optional)

Instructions:

1. Heat olive oil in a large skillet over medium heat. Add minced garlic and cook until fragrant.

2. Add spiralized zucchini noodles to the skillet and sauté for 2-3 minutes, or until noodles are tender but still slightly crisp.

3. Pour marinara sauce over the zucchini noodles and toss to coat.

4. Cook for an additional 2-3 minutes, until heated through.

5. Season with salt and pepper to taste.

6. Serve hot, garnished with vegan Parmesan cheese if desired.

Nutritional info: (per serving)

- Calories: 180

- Protein: 4g

- Carbohydrates: 20g

- Fat: 10g

Chapter 7: Sweet Treats without the Guilt

Vegan Chocolate Chip Cookies

Description: Deliciously soft and chewy chocolate chip cookies made without any animal products.

Preparation time: 15 minutes

Cooking time: 10 minutes

Number of servings: 12 cookies

Ingredients:

- 1/2 cup vegan butter, softened
- 1/2 cup brown sugar

- 1/4 cup granulated sugar

- 1 teaspoon vanilla extract

- 1 1/2 cups all-purpose flour

- 1/2 teaspoon baking soda

- 1/2 teaspoon salt

- 1/4 cup non-dairy milk

- 1 cup vegan chocolate chips

Instructions:

1. Preheat oven to 350°F (175°C) and line a baking sheet with parchment paper.

2. In a large mixing bowl, cream together vegan butter, brown sugar, granulated sugar, and vanilla extract until smooth.

3. In a separate bowl, whisk together flour, baking soda, and salt.

4. Gradually add dry ingredients to the wet ingredients, alternating with non-dairy milk, until fully combined.

5. Fold in vegan chocolate chips.

6. Scoop tablespoon-sized portions of dough onto the prepared baking sheet, leaving space between each cookie.

7. Bake for 10-12 minutes, or until edges are golden brown.

8. Allow cookies to cool on the baking sheet for 5 minutes before transferring to a wire rack to cool completely.

Nutritional info: (per cookie)

- Calories: 180

- Protein: 2g

- Carbohydrates: 25g

- Fat: 8g

Banana Bread

Description: Moist and flavorful banana bread made with ripe bananas and warm spices.

Preparation time: 15 minutes

Cooking time: 1 hour

Number of servings: 10 slices

Ingredients:

- 3 ripe bananas, mashed

- 1/3 cup melted vegan butter or coconut oil

- 1/2 cup brown sugar

- 1 teaspoon vanilla extract

- 1 1/2 cups all-purpose flour

- 1 teaspoon baking soda

- 1/2 teaspoon ground cinnamon

- 1/4 teaspoon salt

Instructions:

1. Preheat oven to 350°F (175°C) and grease a 9x5-inch loaf pan.

2. In a large mixing bowl, combine mashed bananas, melted vegan butter or coconut oil, brown sugar, and vanilla extract.

3. In a separate bowl, whisk together flour, baking soda, cinnamon, and salt.

4. Gradually add dry ingredients to the banana mixture, stirring until just combined.

5. Pour batter into the prepared loaf pan and smooth the top with a spatula.

6. Bake for 50-60 minutes, or until a toothpick inserted into the center comes out clean.

7. Allow banana bread to cool in the pan for 10 minutes before transferring to a wire rack to cool completely.

Nutritional info: (per slice)

- Calories: 200

- Protein: 2g

- Carbohydrates: 30g

- Fat: 8g

Vegan Brownies

Description: Rich and fudgy brownies made without eggs or dairy, perfect for chocolate lovers.

Preparation time: 15 minutes

Cooking time: 25 minutes

Number of servings: 12 brownies

Ingredients:

- 1/2 cup vegan butter, melted

- 1 cup granulated sugar

- 1/4 cup unsweetened cocoa powder

- 1 teaspoon vanilla extract

- 1/2 cup all-purpose flour

- 1/4 teaspoon salt

- 1/4 teaspoon baking powder

- 1/2 cup vegan chocolate chips (optional)

Instructions:

1. Preheat oven to 350°F (175°C) and grease an 8x8-inch baking pan.

2. In a large mixing bowl, whisk together melted vegan butter, granulated sugar, cocoa powder, and vanilla extract until smooth.

3. In a separate bowl, combine flour, salt, and baking powder.

4. Gradually add dry ingredients to the wet ingredients, stirring until just combined.

5. Fold in vegan chocolate chips, if using.

6. Pour batter into the prepared baking pan and spread evenly.

7. Bake for 25-30 minutes, or until a toothpick inserted into the center comes out with moist crumbs.

8. Allow brownies to cool in the pan before slicing into squares.

Nutritional info: (per brownie)

- Calories: 180

- Protein: 2g

- Carbohydrates: 25g

- Fat: 9g

Coconut Bliss Balls

Description: Energy-packed coconut balls made with dates, nuts, and shredded coconut.

Preparation time: 15 minutes

Number of servings: 12 balls

Ingredients:

- 1 cup pitted dates

- 1/2 cup almonds

- 1/2 cup shredded coconut, plus extra for rolling

- 1 tablespoon coconut oil

- 1 tablespoon cocoa powder (optional)

- Pinch of salt

Instructions:

1. In a food processor, blend dates, almonds, shredded coconut, coconut oil, cocoa powder

(if using), and salt until mixture forms a sticky dough.

2. Roll dough into tablespoon-sized balls using your hands.

3. Roll balls in shredded coconut to coat.

4. Place coconut bliss balls in an airtight container and refrigerate for at least 30 minutes before serving.

Nutritional info: (per ball)

- Calories: 90

- Protein: 1g

- Carbohydrates: 12g

- Fat: 5g

Vegan Ice Cream (Various Flavors)

Description: Creamy and decadent ice cream made with non-dairy milk and your favorite flavors.

Preparation time: 10 minutes

Chilling time: 4 hours

Number of servings: 4

Ingredients:

- 2 cups non-dairy milk (such as coconut milk, almond milk, or cashew milk)

- 1/2 cup maple syrup or agave nectar

- 1 teaspoon vanilla extract

- Flavorings of your choice (such as cocoa powder, fruit puree, chopped nuts, or vegan chocolate chips)

Instructions:

1. In a blender, combine non-dairy milk, maple syrup or agave nectar, and vanilla extract.

2. Add flavorings of your choice and blend until smooth.

3. Pour mixture into an ice cream maker and churn according to manufacturer's instructions, usually for about 20-25 minutes.

4. Transfer churned ice cream to a freezer-safe container and freeze for at least 4 hours, or until firm.

5. Allow ice cream to soften for a few minutes at room temperature before serving.

Nutritional info: (per serving)

- Calories: Varies depending on ingredients used

- Protein: Varies depending on ingredients used

- Carbohydrates: Varies depending on ingredients used

- Fat: Varies depending on ingredients used

Fruit Sorbet

Description: Refreshing and fruity sorbet made with fresh fruit and sweetened with a touch of agave nectar.

Preparation time: 10 minutes

Chilling time: 4 hours

Number of servings: 4

Ingredients:

- 2 cups frozen fruit (such as berries, mango, or pineapple)

- 1/4 cup agave nectar or maple syrup

- 2 tablespoons lemon juice

- 1/4 cup water (if needed)

Instructions:

1. In a blender, combine frozen fruit, agave nectar or maple syrup, and lemon juice.

2. Blend until smooth, adding water if necessary to achieve desired consistency.

3. Pour mixture into a freezer-safe container and freeze for at least 4 hours, or until firm.

4. Allow sorbet to soften for a few minutes at room temperature before serving.

Nutritional info: (per serving)

- Calories: Varies depending on fruit used

- Protein: Varies depending on fruit used

- Carbohydrates: Varies depending on fruit used

- Fat: Varies depending on fruit used

Chocolate Avocado Mousse

Description: Creamy and indulgent chocolate mousse made with ripe avocados and cocoa powder.

Preparation time: 10 minutes

Chilling time: 1 hour

Number of servings: 4

Ingredients:

- 2 ripe avocados, peeled and pitted

- 1/4 cup cocoa powder

- 1/4 cup maple syrup or agave nectar

- 1 teaspoon vanilla extract

- Pinch of salt

- Non-dairy milk, if needed

Instructions:

1. In a food processor or blender, combine avocados, cocoa powder, maple syrup or agave nectar, vanilla extract, and salt.

2. Blend until smooth and creamy, adding non-dairy milk if needed to reach desired consistency.

3. Transfer mousse to serving dishes and chill in the refrigerator for at least 1 hour before serving.

4. Garnish with fresh fruit, shredded coconut, or chopped nuts if desired.

    Nutritional info: (per serving)

- Calories: 200

- Protein: 3g

- Carbohydrates: 20g

- Fat: 14g

Veggie Stir-Fry with Tofu

Description: A colorful and flavorful dish packed with vegetables and tofu, stir-fried to perfection.

Preparation time: 15 minutes

Cooking time: 15 minutes

Number of servings: 4

Ingredients:

- 1 block of firm tofu, drained and cubed

- Assorted vegetables (such as bell peppers, broccoli, carrots, and snap peas), sliced

- 3 cloves garlic, minced

- 2 tablespoons soy sauce

- 1 tablespoon sesame oil

- 1 tablespoon vegetable oil

- 1 teaspoon ginger, minced

- Cooked rice or noodles, for serving

Instructions:

1. Heat vegetable oil in a large skillet over medium-high heat. Add tofu cubes and cook

until golden brown on all sides. Remove tofu
from skillet and set aside.

2. In the same skillet, add sesame oil and sauté
garlic and ginger until fragrant.

3. Add sliced vegetables to the skillet and stir-fry
until tender-crisp.

4. Return tofu to the skillet, pour soy sauce over
the tofu and vegetables, and stir to combine.

5. Serve over cooked rice or noodles.

Nutritional info: (per serving)

- Calories: 250

- Protein: 15g

- Carbohydrates: 20g

- Fat: 12g

Vegan Shepherd's Pie

Description: A comforting and hearty dish made with savory lentils and topped with creamy mashed potatoes.

Preparation time: 20 minutes

Cooking time: 40 minutes

Number of servings: 6

Ingredients:

- 1 cup dried lentils

- 2 cups vegetable broth

- 1 onion, diced

- 2 carrots, diced

- 2 cloves garlic, minced

- 1 cup frozen peas

- 2 tablespoons tomato paste

- 1 teaspoon dried thyme

- Salt and pepper, to taste

- 4 large potatoes, peeled and diced

- 1/4 cup non-dairy milk

- 2 tablespoons vegan butter

- 1 tablespoon nutritional yeast (optional)

Instructions:

1. Preheat oven to 375°F (190°C).

2. In a large pot, combine lentils and vegetable broth. Bring to a boil, then reduce heat and simmer for 20 minutes, or until lentils are tender.

3. In a separate skillet, sauté onion, carrots, and garlic until softened.

4. Add cooked lentils, frozen peas, tomato paste, dried thyme, salt, and pepper to the skillet. Cook for an additional 5 minutes.

5. Meanwhile, boil the diced potatoes until fork-tender. Drain and mash with non-dairy milk, vegan butter, nutritional yeast (if using), salt, and pepper.

6. Transfer the lentil mixture to a baking dish and spread mashed potatoes evenly over the top.

7. Bake for 20-25 minutes, or until the mashed potatoes are lightly golden.

Nutritional info: (per serving)

- Calories: 320

- Protein: 12g

- Carbohydrates: 55g

- Fat: 6g

Conclusion

Congratulations on taking the first step toward a more vibrant, plant-based lifestyle! Throughout the pages of this cookbook, you've discovered a wide array of wholesome, nutrient-packed recipes designed to nourish your body and sharpen your mind.

From energizing breakfasts to power you through the morning, to revitalizing lunches that fight the afternoon slump, hearty dinners to replenish you after a long day, and all the snacks, sides and sweet treats in between - you now have a wholefood culinary toolkit to help you feel your best.

Beyond just the recipes themselves, you've also learned tips for stocking a plant-based kitchen, meal prepping for convenience, boosting nutrition with simple ingredient swaps and cooking techniques, and so much more. Armed with this knowledge, you can continue to get creative and craft delicious plant-based dishes tailored to your tastes.

Remember, this way of eating is all about progress, not perfection. Even small steps like incorporating more fresh produce, whole grains, legumes, nuts and seeds into your routine can make a big difference in how you look and feel each day. Stay focused on nourishing your body and mind, while allowing yourself flexibility to make this lifestyle work for you.

We hope this book has ignited your passion for plant-based cooking and self-care. Stick with it, keep exploring new recipes and ingredients, and trust that every wholesome bite is an investment in your overall health, clarity and vitality for years to come. Here's to a lifetime of feeling energized!